HIT BY AN ICEBERG

Printed in Victoria, Canada

National Library of Canada Cataloguing in Publication

Freedman, Janet
Hit by an iceberg : coping with disability mid-career / Janet Freedman, Marie Howes.
Includes bibliographical references and index.
ISBN 1-4120-0211-7
1. People with disabilities--Services for--Canada. 2. People with disabilities--Legal status, laws, etc.--Canada. I. Howes, Marie II. Title.
HV1559.C3F735 2003   362.4'0971   C2003-901979-9

TRAFFORD

This book was published *on-demand* in cooperation with Trafford Publishing. On-demand publishing is a unique process and service of making a book available for retail sale to the public taking advantage of on-demand manufacturing and Internet marketing. **On-demand publishing** includes promotions, retail sales, manufacturing, order fulfilment, accounting and collecting royalties on behalf of the author.

Suite 6E, 2333 Government St., Victoria, B.C. V8T 4P4, CANADA
Phone   250-383-6864   Toll-free 1-888-232-4444 (Canada & US)
Fax   250-383-6804   E-mail   sales@trafford.com
Web site www.trafford.com TRAFFORD PUBLISHING IS A DIVISION OF TRAFFORD HOLDINGS LTD.
Trafford Catalogue #03-0579   www.trafford.com/robots/03-0579.html

10   9   8   7   6   5   4   3   2

HIT BY AN ICEBERG

Coping with Disability in Mid-Career

Janet Freedman and Marie Howes

Trafford

This book is dedicated to

François Dansereau and Vincent Dansereau,
whose rescue of Janet allowed her to
live and write this book;

And to

A. Gavin Clark
and
Jonathan Freedman
and
Rachel Freedman

With love and appreciation

MH and JF

CONTENTS

DISCLAIMER

While every effort has been made to provide an accurate overview of the topics and programs described in this book, readers are cautioned that since laws and regulations frequently change, they must consult with reputable professional advisors to obtain up-to-date information and advice for their particular situation. The material provided in this book is of a general nature and intended for information purposes only.

The authors cannot be responsible for actions readers may take based on information contained in this book, nor can they be responsible for any errors or omissions contained in the text.

Specialized accounting, financial, insurance, investment, legal, and tax advisors should be retained to assist in overall planning for individuals and their families.

ACKNOWLEDGEMENTS

At the outset, we wish to acknowledge and thank all those friends and colleagues who rallied and helped Janet's business survive the first year of her disability. Special thanks are due to JoAnne Anderson, Jaquelyn Bradshaw and Diane Miller. Thanks also to Carole Aronovitch for her ongoing support.

As the book began to take shape, we gathered more and more information and encouragement. Thanks to all the people who shared their stories with us and who provided invaluable insight into living with disabilities. Thanks also to the numerous staff and friends at the Toronto Rehabilitation Institute, Lyndhurst Centre. Many people working with people with disabilities at organizations from coast to coast to coast shared their insights with us for which we are very grateful.

We want to express our appreciation to the Easter Seals / March of Dimes National Council for their support and endorsement of this book, especially Michele Sharp.

Many busy professionals in the health care, legal, financial, insurance, investment, and publishing worlds took the time to give us advice, information and support, for which we are very grateful: Jane Baker, Barbara Carter, Margaret Hall, Sandra Foster, Carien Jutting, Irene Lenney, Larry Marshall LL.B., Mary Matusi, Kent McKelvey, Ian Parker, Arthur Rosenbaum, John Rousseau, Dr. Marie Roy, Douglas Strelshik LL.B., Glorianne Stromberg, Catherine Thompson, Dr. Murray Waldman.

Thanks also to Bonnie Heath for copy editing; John Zehethofer for our cover design; and Barbara Webber and John Wild, photographer, for making our photographic selves look good!

All the mistakes are solely our own—we will make corrections in our next edition.

JF and MH,
Toronto, August 2003

FOREWORD

"Nothing in life is to be feared, it is only to be understood. Now is the time to understand more, so that we may fear less." Marie Curie (1867 - 1934)

Every once in a while, a book comes along that is both timely and long overdue. **Hit by an Iceberg: Coping with Disability in Mid-Career** is such a book. An individual's sudden disability, caused by an accident or adult onset illness, is devastating for both the person with a disability and their family, friends and advisors. Where do caregivers/legal representatives turn for information and guidance? What services and support systems are out there for a person with a disability? How can they access all the services and financial help to which they may be entitled? When do they need to consult professional advisors such as lawyers and investment managers? Where do they find these advisors and how do they evaluate these services? Until now, there has not been a ready reference guide to help individuals, families or professional advisors and caregivers.

The authors have firsthand knowledge of the information necessary to cope with sudden disability. Janet's spinal cord was partially severed in a fall on April 14, 2000 (88 years to the day of the sinking of the Titanic). Marie and her husband held Power of Attorney for Janet. The long and complex process which brought Janet from near paralysis to recovery inspired this book. During rehabilitation, Janet observed that many disabled people and their families and friends were unsure of what they could or should be doing to ensure that maximum financial, lifestyle and legal benefits were in place for the family member with the disability.

Professional advisors in the insurance, investment and financial planning fields need such a reference for training new advisors and for helping clients who become disabled. Health care and legal professionals, from administrators and advocates, to doctors and other health care professionals, to social workers and lawyers, will also welcome such a resource. Factual information and illustrations from many interviews and case histories help people understand how to handle disability situations.

As Marie Curie said, the more we understand, the more empowered we become. Knowledge is power. With knowledge, we can take preventive measures; but we will also know what to do if a disability does occur.

Congratulations to Janet and Marie for putting all this information together.

Bill Mates
Chair, National Affairs and Public Education Committee
Easter Seals / March of Dimes National Council
Toronto, Ontario.
March 2003

PROLOGUE

Marie's story

It was mid-morning on April 14, 2000 when the phone rang. It was JoAnne Anderson.

Have you heard yet? Janet has fallen at home, down her front steps. She trapped her head between her front stairs and those next door. She was conscious when the neighbours found her. She's in Toronto Western Hospital with a C6 spinal fracture. It's serious. She may be paralyzed. Rachel thinks you have power of attorney—do you?"

Frankly, I didn't remember. "I know we're the executors of Janet's will when she dies, but I think she said some other friends had P of A; but perhaps that was for Personal Care."

Very soon after that telephone call, Rachel, Janet's 18-year-old daughter phoned. "I think you and Gavin have power of attorney for my mum. Do you have the documents? Do you know where they are?" I said that I didn't—which is not unusual since such documents are not usually delivered to the appointed person until they must act.

So—where were the documents? Janet was now medicated and sedated, unable to speak. Places to look: Safety deposit box—but which bank? And where was the key? Lawyer's office? Tried there but no copy on file. Home lock box or file? Yes! When we reviewed the papers, my husband, Gavin, and I, were indeed named as joint holders of power of attorney for Janet Freedman.

It was the beginning of an experience that we will not easily forget; nor do we hope ever to repeat. It was an adventure into *terra incognita*. Just as the Arctic explorers had to navigate through dangerous icebergs, we discovered some initially invisible legal, financial and emotional shoals through which we had to pass. A disability is like an iceberg: it appears to be of a certain measurable dimension. But the reality is that 80% of its impact is hidden after the initial encounter. Yet most Canadians have little idea of what devastating effects a disability can have on a loved one or friend or colleague. And they underrate the consequences for themselves as bystanders, caregivers, or legal representatives. This apart from what the person with the disability must face.

This book is an attempt to provide a practical, functional framework for relatives, professional financial planners, lawyers and other professionals, colleagues and friends who are faced with helping someone cope with disability. We have focused on the effects of disability arising from a sudden incident or illness during peoples' working years or mid-career. We will not discuss disability in old age or in retirement.

This book is also a call to arms—strong arms, caring arms—to challenge the very real problems associated with dealing with a disability in Canada. We've come a long way—but there are many islands of apathy and outdated laws and rules, frozen by tradition. We need change if people with disabilities are to function to the best of their abilities in Canadian society.

CHAPTER 1

THE TIP OF THE ICEBERG

Death is mortality; a finality. Disability is morbidity; a possibility of harm.
Death is inevitable; it comes ultimately to us all.
Disability is a probability; it is a random selection that could happen to anyone.

A Statistics Canada report, "A Profile of Disability in Canada, 2001," shows that about 3.4 million Canadians over age 15 have some degree of recognized disability. Their situations range from *mild* (5% of the total identified) to *very severe* (2% of the total identified). But in cold figures, these 3.4 million people represent one in seven, or 15% of Canadian adults. Of these, some 480,000 have *very severe* disabilities, whereas about 914,400 have *severe* disabilities. That is, 6% of adult Canadians over age 15 have some form of *severe* or *very severe* disability.

Statistics Canada's 1996 study of "Disability-Free Life Expectancy" shows that males with a life expectancy of 76 years have, statistically, a disability-free life expectancy of 69 years. In other words, they may suffer some form of disability for 7 years of their lives, on average.

For females, with a life expectancy of 81 years, the disability-free life expectancy is 70 years, or 11 years of potential disability, on average.

Between your age now and age 65, you will earn thousands of dollars, perhaps millions, if you work until retirement. For example, if you are earning a gross income of $3,000 per month and are age 35, you will earn a total of $1,712,714 by age 65, assuming 3% annual pay increases over that time. If you are age 45 and earn $5,000 per month, then by age 65 you will earn $1,612,222 assuming 3% annual pay raises.

1

But if disability interrupts your income flow, your lifestyle and that of your family could change dramatically unless you have ways to replace your income. This is where government, employer and private disability programs come into play. Your own investments also form part of the "repair" package. There is, however, more to a disability than money; there are other adjustments that have to be made. The iceberg runs deep beneath the surface.

Disability can range from a broken arm to a severed spinal cord; from post-traumatic stress disorder to chronic fatigue syndrome to disability caused by a stroke, or to diseases such as multiple sclerosis or Lou Gehrig's disease. Disability can be caused by an accident or a risky lifestyle, or it can be the result of a disease—which in turn can move slowly or rapidly. It is random in nature unless there is a genetic or lifestyle link. There is a greater risk of disability than there is of death for those under age 65. Yet few people appreciate the extent of the risk.

In disability cases, time is the enemy. An accident victim needs immediate care to reduce the risk of further trauma or injury. The person with a debilitating disease is at the mercy of time if the disease is progressive and no cure or treatment is available.

But time can also be the healer. Bones mend. Stress can be relieved with therapy or medications. Some people, though, never recover. Many—perhaps most—never regain 100% of pre-disability function.

What Life Factors Are Affected By A Disability?

When a disability occurs, many aspects of life are thrown into turmoil. These are some of the most important:

- Physical and/or mental changes: the disability may affect a person's physical movement and bodily functions and/or their mental capacities and perceptions.

- Financial issues: the disability may cause income disruption, possible depletion of assets, indebtedness, inability to borrow, forced sale of home.
- Legal issues: incapacity may trigger power of attorney, decisions being made by others, or the provincial rules concerning competency under Public Trustee or Official Guardian legislation may be triggered if there is no one holding power of attorney for the person with the disability.
- Housing changes: the person's home may no longer be suitable for them, or they may no longer be able to pay the mortgage and may have to sell the house.
- Psychological factors: the person may be unable to cope emotionally with his or her new situation; relatives, colleagues or friends may be equally unable to accept the situation without counselling; children may be affected and may not have the capacity to deal with the changes to their routines.
- Bureaucratic imposition: local, provincial, and federal policies govern the type and extent of financial help, care, services, and facilities a person with a disability may receive and when they may start; private or employer insurance plans impose restrictions before payments are made.
- Taxation provisions: if certain conditions are met, people with disabilities and their families may be entitled to special claims on their tax returns.
- Frustration factors: the person with the disability may be frustrated by being unable to communicate his or her wishes; those holding power of attorney must act for the person with the disability—even if some instructions seem impractical or counterproductive.

Disability: The Triggering Event

Disability is one of the "Four Dreadful D's"—those events in life that are dreaded or feared: Downsizing, Divorce, Disability, Death.

How do people facing disability react to their altered lives? Their reactions are similar to those reported by people who are bereaved. There are several responses in common:

- Disbelief
- Anger
- Bargaining
- Avoidance
- Depression
- Acceptance

The response of family and loved ones may be similar, or there may also be an irrational response on their part. The family member or loved one may simply exit the scene entirely—and leave the person with the disability to cope on his or her own. Sometimes the irrational response is to become manic—cleaning the home, trying to make things "perfect" since the person with the disability is now no longer "perfect" or whole.

But most human beings are amazingly adaptive: they confront their situation, no matter how unforeseen or unpleasant it may be, and they try to make the best of it.

Dr. Murray Waldman, Director of Rehabilitation at St. John's Hospital, Toronto, has thought a lot about disability and how it fits into the Canadian medicare system. Here are some of his observations, considered over the course of his career in medicine and rehabilitation.

The medical model is based entirely on diagnosis and treatment. When you go into an acute care hospital, the process is, "What's wrong with you? Can we treat it?" Most medical schools focus 90% on diagnosis, 10% on treatment. This is a fine model, but disability and rehabilitation are not concerned with diagnosis. People come to us already diagnosed, and as far as the medical system goes, already treated.

But disability and rehabilitation is the difference between *getting* better and *feeling* better. Disability is, in effect, a *functional* diagnosis.... You become disabled when you can't do something that you used to be able to do before whatever it was happened. At the end of the day, it comes down to: "I am disabled because I can't do today what I could do yesterday." Then you ask yourself whether it's transient or permanent; is it going to get worse; is it going to get better; is it going to stay the same? If you have ALS, it's going to be progressive; if you've had a stroke you are likely to get better—maybe not 100%, but you may improve. If you've had an amputation, it's going to stay the same. Rehabilitation doesn't consist of a return *of* function—its aim is to return a person *to* function.

The sad thing is that we have a two-tier health care system.... Rich people get better care without having to pay extra. For example, if you're a wealthy matron and you need a pacemaker, you will get the $5,000 version rather than the $500 version. It's up to your physician which one you get. If you or your family knows that St. John's or another fine rehab unit exists, the chances are you'll demand and get good rehab. If you don't know about it, you could well be sent home to struggle on your own. There are huge inequities in the system. The wealthy don't pay for it; they just have access to it. There are a lot of resources out there where one can access information and find out what is available. You have to know what to ask.

Governments have come to believe that they can run General Hospital like they run General Motors. There's a huge difference—General Motors can tell you within a nickel how much it costs to make a Buick by costing out every nut and bolt. General Hospital can, if they really work at it, tell you exactly how much it cost to fix your neck. The difference is General Motors can tell you what that Buick is worth and how much value has been added by putting everything together, but how much more is Janet worth with the repaired neck than she was without it? There is no way of putting a value on that. General Motors can stop producing an unprofitable car. The population will not accept ceasing to treat 'unprofitable' health care.

SOURCES OF INFORMATION

Statistics Canada Web site: www.statcan.ca

CHAPTER 2

WHEN THE ICEBERG HITS

Janet's story

The sun was shining, the birds were singing and, apart from the stress that income tax season brings to those whose livelihood depends on preparing personal tax returns, April 14 was a lovely spring day. As I went hurtling through the air, the thought that went through my mind was "I knew I should have taken two trips to the car." I was late for a meeting with a client and had my arms full of bags of tax returns. Then I missed a step outside my front door and fell....

I landed on my head, trapped between my front steps and the neighbours' front steps, my neck snapped back, my windpipe blocked. I couldn't breathe. I couldn't move any part of my body. I couldn't call out for help. I was scared.

But I had noticed that my neighbours were loading up their truck to go to work, and I knew they would see me when they came out—I hoped that would be soon. It was. They immediately realized the seriousness of the situation and, after one of them called 911, lifted me vertically up supporting my neck and then laid me down horizontally on the path. As they lifted me out, I gasped for air and said, "Thank you, thank you, thank you." Another neighbour came over with a blanket. The first to arrive, as usual in Toronto, was the fire department.

Then the ambulance came. The police arrived and wanted to know what happened and whether I wanted my daughter to be notified. I said no. Another neighbour offered to come with me to the hospital. I was moved gently onto a backboard, my neck stabilized, and off we went to the hospital with sirens blaring. Ambulances are not the most comfortable mode of transportation, and I was in some pain. I could feel my left arm (which felt broken), but nothing else below my neck except that my legs felt as if they were in a sitting position—bent at the knee. They took me to St. Michael's hospital first, where I was again questioned by police. They wanted to know whether I had consumed alcohol or illegal drugs, whether I had blacked out or been pushed, whether I was wearing high heels. (The answer was no to all the above!) All the way through and until I had surgery, I kept cracking jokes. It must be part of the shock reaction.

When someone is injured or suffers a medical emergency, the coping mechanisms start with emergency response teams. The initial response to a 911 call may be handled by the police or by the fire department; they in turn may call for an ambulance.

Once at hospital, the medical system takes over. Following an accident, the emergency department medical team first determines the extent and seriousness of the injury, the procedures needed to stabilize the patient, and the speed at which certain procedures must be administered.

If the disability is one diagnosed by a doctor during a regular examination rather than in an emergency situation such as an accident, heart attack, or stroke, then treatment proceeds in a more orderly and planned manner.

Either way, the Canadian health care system's objective is to treat patients effectively and efficiently— as quickly and with as short a stay in a medical facility as possible and at the lowest possible cost. Where appropriate outpatient care is available, that is the treatment delivery method of choice.

Patients are treated under the rules of the medical system as set out by their province of residence, since health care is a provincial responsibility. Each province covers certain basic procedures, but not necessarily others.

The theory is that every Canadian receives high quality, essentially equivalent care across the country. The reality is that outside major centres there are fewer facilities and even fewer specialists. This is a serious problem if a person suffers a traumatic injury, which, for example, requires neurological intervention. In cases of spinal cord injury, the sooner steroids are administered, the less swelling there is and the greater the chance the patient will avoid complete paralysis. But if there is a delay in transporting the patient from the site of their injury to a properly equipped medical facility, then the patient's recovery may be compromised.

WHAT THE FAMILY OR RESPONSIBLE PERSON NEEDS TO KNOW

Legal Matters: Consent To Treatment

Before the medical professionals can begin systematic care of the patient, there are certain legal niceties that must be followed. Each hospital in the provincial medical system normally requires the consent of the patient before procedures begin. If patients are incapable of giving their consent, then that consent must be given by the next of kin or the patient's legal representative (See Chapter 3: "Who Can Act for You? Powers of Attorney".) Consent does not have to be in writing—it may be given orally as happened in Janet's case. Of course, in emergency situations when no one is available to consent, treatment goes ahead regardless of consent.

Immediately upon arrival at the hospital, the doctor asked me if I consented to treatment, in the presence of a second doctor, as they were wheeling me down the hall. When I responded that I didn't really have any choice, did I? they took that as consent to treatment. But later on, when I was very ill with pneumonia and was incapable of giving consent, my daughter was asked to give consent to an alternative treatment.

Who are *next of kin*? If the patient is married, then the spouse is next of kin; if there is no spouse, then adult children (over age 18) are next of kin; if the patient is a minor child, then the parent is the next of kin. In the case of an unmarried adult with no adult dependents, the holder of power of attorney for that person can be called upon. Of course, if no next of kin or legal representative can be found, care is still provided and the province takes responsibility for the person through the Attorney General's department.

In the emergency room, the objective is to stabilize the patient so that long-term treatment decisions can be made. This is where the legal representative or next of kin plays an important role. Often there are a number of ways of treating disabling injuries or illnesses. The patient may have certain views as to what procedures are, or are not, acceptable to him or her. The next of kin can consider the patient's wishes and interpret them to the medical staff. Indeed, the next of kin may be asked to consent to new or experimental procedures if the patient is unable to give consent or make decisions for himself or herself.

The next of kin can give consent for medical procedures orally (especially in an emergency situation) or in writing. If permission to follow certain procedures is given in writing, the hospital staff will provide forms that must be *signed off* by the patient or the patient's representative. The patient may also give oral consent with a witness present.

When consent to treatment is given, it is "blanket consent" and covers all procedures that may have to be taken if unexpected conditions or circumstances arise, especially during surgery.

Those who do *not* consent to certain procedures, such as blood transfusions, must state this when agreeing to other procedures. (With such prohibitions, some surgeons may elect not to proceed with particular procedures.)

If the disabling accident or illness proves fatal, the patient may want certain organs to be donated to others or to a medical research facility. This is why it is important to have a donor card filled out and attached to a driver's licence or otherwise have organ donor instructions filed with medical staff. Family and friends should be aware of the person's wishes in this regard.

Setting up power of attorney documents is an important preventive measure that people can take to ensure their wishes are followed should a disability occur. This is covered in detail in the following chapter, but briefly, *Power of Attorney for Personal Care* (and *Power of Attorney for Property, Financial and Legal Affairs*) are legal documents that allow a named person(s), other than the *donor* (person who gives the authority), to act on behalf of the donor, just as if the donor were present and able to act on his or her own behalf. The power given under Power of Attorney for Personal Care or Advanced Health Care Directive is a form of consent that allows the person who receives the authority to decide on medical or personal care options for the donor. The authority is exercised by the named person in cases when the donor is incapable of making decisions on his or her own behalf, for example, if the person is in a coma or is unable to speak because of injury or other medical condition.

What Happens In The Hospital In A Disability Case?

If the disabling accident or event is severe and requires high-level medical intervention, then the patient will most likely be in the intensive care unit (ICU) for a period of time. The ICU has the most nurses and doctors on duty compared with other departments in the hospital. The patients in this setting are in critical condition and must be watched constantly.

Once patients have been stabilized, they will then be moved to an acute care unit of the hospital. This unit still provides intensive nursing care, but not at the same level as the ICU.

The Hospital Setting

A patient in an ICU observes several factors, such as:
- Constant noise
- Bright lights
- Administration of heavy-duty medications that may provoke adverse reactions
- Few nurses available to provide optimum care because of cutbacks in the system

The shortage of nurses means that family and friends may be called upon to assist in the patient's recovery. Indeed, if at all possible, experience recommends that anyone in an ICU have family and friends take round-the-clock shifts at the bedside. When in an ICU, the patient is typically on a ventilator and/or unconscious. Nurses are not always on hand when a patient becomes agitated. In these circumstances, patients need advocates.

The medical staff will be asking the patient many questions. Communication can sometimes be a problem. Some hints for dealing with these difficulties.
- Friends or family who can lip-read can be a great help to the medical staff and to the patient who cannot speak normally, especially if the patient has had a tracheotomy.
- Patients on ventilators will be able to communicate only with their hands and/or eyes.

The noise level in some hospital wards can be very upsetting to patients, especially those who are unable to speak and voice their annoyance. Commented one patient:

If I had one piece of advice for improving patient care, I would tell people caring for patients coming out of anesthesia to "SHUT UP!"

Janet's story

The radio that was blaring non-stop in the ICU seemed to play Madonna singing "Don't Cry for me Argentina" over and over and over again. Now, whenever I hear that song, I want to do what I couldn't do in the hospital—SCREAM! And sometimes I do! Nurses and caregivers need to realize that this type of music, as well as chattering about the fight they had with their husband/boyfriend/children/parents that day, are not conversations that patients want to hear. And conversations held within earshot are often incorporated into the delirium and hallucinations that many ICU patients experience.

Dealing With Inquiries About The Patient

The next of kin or personal representative will also have to deal with inquiries about the patient's condition. Often, people will want to send flowers or other gifts. Some hints on handling such inquiries:

- No flowers or gifts are permitted in the ICU; even some acute care units restrict flowers depending upon the patient's condition.
- Visiting in the ICU is normally restricted to immediate family; acute care units also have visiting restrictions. Of course, the family and patient can also restrict visitors.
- If the patient has an answering machine or automatic messaging service on their phone, the family should compose a brief message to callers that briefly states the facts of the patient's condition and the patient's and family's wishes regarding flowers or visits.

- Suggest that concerned friends or colleagues may want to wait before sending flowers or gifts to a time when the patient will be able to appreciate them.
- Sometimes, the patient would like to have a special kind of food. If permitted by the patient's doctor, suggest that friends might bring that instead of flowers!
- Family and other caregivers should not feel guilty about turning down visitors if the patient doesn't wish it, or if the connection is remote.

SOURCES OF INFORMATION

From the Ashes of My Dreams, Ed Smith. Flanker Press, 2002
A personal account of adventures and misadventures in hospitals and rehabilitation centres in Newfoundland and Ontario, following a motor vehicle accident.

CHAPTER 3

WHO CAN ACT FOR YOU? POWERS OF ATTORNEY

Janet's story

The critical issue with a spinal cord injury is to get treatment as soon as possible—treatment that consists of large doses of steroids to prevent swelling of the spinal cord. It is this swelling that does most of the damage. I was put on steroids almost immediately. There were X-rays, a CAT scan and an MRI. Much of the time I was in a haze of unreality and pain. That evening I was transferred to Toronto Western Hospital, which handles most spinal cord injury cases in the Toronto region. Saturday morning I had surgery that lasted five hours or so.

The doctor put one word on the diagnosis page of my disability application: paralysis. My attorneys feared the worst—that I would have quadriplegia.

Ultimately, the diagnosis was Brown-Sequard syndrome. This is normally seen in patients stabbed in the neck or with gunshot wounds to the neck. It also means that only one side of the spinal cord is severely damaged. Since the spinal cord can reroute messages around the site of injury, the prognosis is more hopeful. What had actually happened was that the sixth cervical vertebra was crushed. (All mammals have seven cervical vertebra, counted by starting at the top of the neck downwards.) This was then replaced using a bone graft from my right hip. A titanium plate was used to connect the fifth to seventh vertebrae. The surgery was done from the front of my neck.

A "halo" was then attached to my head, which itself attaches to a rigid plastic vest, lined with sheepskin, that extends to the waist. The halo is a metal contraption that looks a lot more uncomfortable than it actually is. It weighs about 10 pounds and is screwed into the skull with nasty looking screws—two above the ears and two in the forehead. This form of traction, which immobilizes the whole upper body, has to be worn for at least three months—sometimes longer—to give the bones a chance to heal and fuse. My head was shaved, for which I apparently gave my consent. In retrospect it was sensible, as it is very hard to wash hair or keep it tidy and unmatted with the halo on.

From the time of my surgery, I remember very little clearly. Things became very confused in my mind. I developed pneumonia after the surgery and as a result, spent three weeks in the Intensive Care Unit (ICU). As I was on a ventilator, I was unable to speak or communicate with the nurses or my family. Paralysis meant I couldn't write either. Heavy sedation led to hallucinations and delirium.

WHO CAN ACT FOR YOU WHEN YOU CANNOT?

In the provinces that operate under Common Law principles, that is, all provinces except Quebec, the document known as power of attorney gives the authority for someone to act on behalf of a person who is incapacitated (by an accident or debilitating illness) and who cannot legally act on his or her own behalf. In Quebec, the equivalent document is known as a mandate. Because there are a number of legal and technical terms involved in the discussion of who can act for you, there is a short glossary of terms at the end of the chapter.

The person who gives the power to act is called the *donor*, because he or she is granting or "donating" the power. The person who takes responsibility for the donor is called the *attorney* (hence, power of attorney). This attorney should not be confused with a donor's lawyer. The *attorney* in *power of attorney* is simply a trusted individual whom the donor has selected, and is probably not a lawyer. This person is also sometimes referred to as the *holder*, that is, the holder of the power of attorney. Of course, before granting a power of attorney, you should check with the potential holder to be sure that this person is willing to become an attorney, because the position does carry potential liability in relation to the donor and the beneficiaries of the donor's estate.

Power of attorney is an important part of defensive planning for all adults. Many people assume that if they have written a will, then their executor/trustee can take charge of their affairs if they become disabled. This is not so. An executor/trustee can assume control over an individual's financial and legal affairs only after the death of the *testator* (person writing the will), not during the testator's lifetime.

The procedure for managing your affairs if you become incapacitated is to set up a power of attorney document *before* you suffer incapacity. That incapacity may be the result of an accident, onset of mental disability or from another cause. The document must set up an *enduring* or *continuing* power of attorney. This means that the wording in the document must allow the document to be valid when you, the *donor* (person granting the power), become incapacitated and the *attorney* (person holding the power) is required to act. This is a legal nicety, which is one more reason to have a lawyer or notary draft up not only wills, but also powers of attorney. They know the right words!

Once granted, a power of attorney does not have an "expiry date" except when one of the following takes place:

- The donor dies, or
- The holder of power of attorney dies and does not have an executor/trustee, or
- The donor gives written notice of revocation to the holder and/or
- The donor notifies all persons with whom the holder of the power of attorney had dealings on the donor's behalf, that the power of attorney is now

revoked. This notice may or may not be in writing, or,

- The donor deliberately physically destroys all copies in order to revoke the power of attorney.

Power of attorney comes in two forms in most provinces:

- Power of Attorney for Property, Financial, and Legal Affairs
- Power of Attorney for Personal Care (sometimes called a Living Will)

POWER OF ATTORNEY FOR PROPERTY, FINANCIAL, AND LEGAL AFFAIRS

The most common form of power of attorney is Power of Attorney for Property, Financial, and Legal Affairs, (usually shortened to Power of Attorney for Property or Financial Power of Attorney). This means that the attorney can manage the financial, legal, investment, and ordinary cash flow matters of the person who has been incapacitated. It is a power that confers virtually all the same rights, responsibilities, and capacities the individual donor had while he or she was able to act on his or her own behalf. (A holder of a power of attorney cannot write a new will or change the existing will of the donor.)

Note that Continuing Power of Attorney for Property comes into effect immediately. In other words, there is no requirement that the person in fact be incapacitated before the authority vests in the attorney. The donor must give a specific directive saying that the power of attorney can come into effect only if the donor is incapacitated and that the incapacity must be verified by medical professionals. Otherwise, the authority is created, and can be exercised, when the document is signed. (See 'The triggering event' later in this chapter.)

Choosing Your Attorneys for Property

Who will act for you if you cannot? Who should you choose to hold power of attorney on your behalf?

Some guidelines:

- More than one person can be named to hold power of attorney on your behalf. If possible, it is advisable to name at least two people to act jointly as attorneys. The reason? The work can be onerous and time consuming. (With three named attorneys, there can be a tie-breaker in the event of a disagreement.)
- The person(s) chosen to hold power of attorney must be those whom you trust absolutely. This document confers enormous power on the attorneys. They can do anything that you could do, were you capable of acting on your own behalf, with the exceptions discussed above.
- Ideal attorneys are financially responsible people: they understand how to deal with financial institutions, with financial transactions such as mortgages, loans, investments and regular household accounting.

In the case of married couples in stable marriages, usually each spouse gives the other power of attorney. It is also possible to make an adult child (or children) a co-attorney or an alternate attorney. Of course, non-family members can be named as attorneys also. Problems arise when adult children are appointed attorneys if they are warring among themselves, or if they do not have the parent's best interests at heart. Avoid appointing children in these circumstances. One way around these problems may be to appoint two children jointly so that both signatures are always required.

You should also name *alternate* attorneys in the event that your chosen attorney(s) cannot act for some reason. This is especially important for married couples: if both happen to be in an accident and are injured, then alternate attorneys must act for either or both of them. Alternates should be named in all power of attorney documents since there may be times when a named attorney is unable to act on behalf of the donor. By naming alternate(s), the donor is able to determine who will act as attorney, no matter what the circumstances.

It's also preferable, for convenience, to have attorneys who live in the same city or province. If there is a sizeable estate, at least two attorneys should be named. This is especially important if there is no surviving spouse, or if the spouse or other beneficiaries are not very familiar with money management or the management of an estate. (The term *estate* simply means the assets and legal and financial obligations of the donor, that is, the person granting the power of attorney.)

If the donor has a business, it is advisable to have a power of attorney that notes that fact and that specifically allows the attorneys to act in regard to that business (or that specifies who is to act concerning the business if the attorneys are not the same for personal and business affairs.)

Power of attorney should not be given lightly: it is a powerful document. You must trust the person or persons to whom you are giving such authority.

The holder of the power of attorney is in a position of trust: if the holder mismanages the donor's affairs, then fraud charges can be laid. It is essential for the holder of the power of attorney to keep good records.

The Triggering Event

It is worth repeating that a Continuing Power of Attorney for Property comes into effect immediately when it is signed *unless* the document says it comes into effect only in certain circumstances. The event that gives rise to the use of power of attorney is called the *triggering event,* and it is defined by the donor. What event or condition has to occur before the power of attorney can be used? Is it mental incapacity or physical impairment as determined by a physician or specialist? How is the attorney's right to act verified? Is it an application to the donor's lawyer accompanied by a doctor's certificate? When you draw up your powers of attorney documents, you must answer these questions. Get qualified legal advice.

Extent of the Power being Granted

A key consideration in naming a power of attorney is the extent of the power you, as the donor, wish to grant. Is the definition of power broad enough to permit effective action, yet narrow enough to allow for the constraints that you may wish to place on the attorneys? The objective is to allow the attorneys to act in a timely manner, yet prevent fraud from occurring at the hands of unscrupulous holders of the power of attorney.

The power granted under the power of attorney document can be *broad* or *general*, or *limited*. Obviously, a broad or general power of attorney allows the holder of the power to act on a wide range of matters. A limited power may restrict the holder to certain aspects of your financial and legal affairs: for example, the holder may be able to deal only with your investment portfolio or only with matters of real estate. The donor states the limits in the power of attorney document. It is preferable that there not be too many restrictions on the attorney—otherwise, they may not be able to act quickly or effectively.

Typical powers granted to attorneys include the right to:
- Deposit and withdraw money in bank accounts
- Buy and sell stocks, bonds and mutual funds
- File tax returns
- Sell and buy real estate
- Make charitable donations

- Make loans
- Manage an existing business in which the donor participated

Compensation for the Holder of Power of Attorney

All expenses incurred by the attorney in the course of managing your estate if you are incapacitated can be reimbursed. These expenses must, however, be reasonable and conform to guidelines in the power of attorney granted or in provincial regulations. Examples of reasonable expenses are postage, photocopying, kilometres or mileage to the bank.

Annual compensation, as a trustee fee for the holder of power of attorney, can be set out in the power of attorney document or is estimated based on provincial or Common Law principles. Typically, it can be one-half of one per cent of the assets under management.

If There is No Power of Attorney in Place

If you do not have a Power of Attorney for Property in place, each province has its own set of rules as to how a disabled or incapacitated person's affairs are to be managed. The provincial Public Trustee or Official Guardian's office assumes control of your estate. The province takes charge of your finances: paying bills, even selling assets if necessary. In such cases, the Office of the Public Trustee in the provincial Attorney General's Office will assume control over your property, legal and financial affairs after a period of time has elapsed. (See chart for provincial details.) The Trustee's office must be notified if there is no valid Power of Attorney for Property and if a person's disability or incapacity continues for a period of time. This means that family or friends must follow certain procedures if they wish to manage the person's affairs when there is no power of attorney set up.

The province wants to protect you as the patient or incapacitated person from financial and legal hazards. This is why the Public Trustee/Official Guardian's office exists. Anyone who wishes to apply to take over the responsibility for managing the affairs of an incapacitated person (if there is no holder of power of attorney) must apply to the Office of the Public Trustee for permission to do so. (See below.)

The Office of the Public Trustee/Official Guardian may not necessarily manage your living estate in the way that you wish. If you do not set up powers of attorney, you lose your right to have your assets managed as you would have liked.

Some Additional Points about Power of Attorney

- Joint bank accounts can come under the control of the Office of the Public Trustee if it feels such control is necessary. That is, that share of a joint bank account that is in the name of the incapacitated person may be frozen by the Public Trustee's office.
- If the matrimonial home must be sold and the incapacitated person has a share in that home, then it may be that the courts will have to authorize a sale in lieu of the signature of one of the spouses (assuming there is no holder of a power of attorney to complete the transaction).
- Power of attorney forms filled in by bank customers are valid only at that bank (and at all branches of that bank).
- People over age 18 who own property and assets should have power of attorney documents drawn up or have a mandate prepared in the Province of Quebec.

The Single Person and Power of Attorney

If you are single with no spouse, choosing attorneys can be more of a problem. You must have absolute trust and confidence in the person you choose to be the holder of the power. If single people do not know anyone who fits that description, then they must rely on their provincial public trustee's office and its rules governing the administration of assets of incapacitated persons. It is better to have no attorney at all than to have one who is untrustworthy or incompetent.

An alternative is to name a trust company to assume the role of attorney. You must pay compensation to the trust company for such services. The formula for such compensation is contained in the agreement with the trust company when the documents are drawn up.

If someone wishes to have administration of the single person's assets (estate) upon disability, that person must apply to the provincial Attorney General's office of the Public Trustee or Official Guardian, for permission to do so. Many provinces now require a bond to be posted and a written plan submitted for how the assets will be administered before authority is given to a would-be attorney, even if that applicant is a family member.

The holder of a power of attorney is in a fiduciary role, that is, a position of trust. A holder has an obligation to act ethically on behalf of the donor for whom they are acting. Funds managed and spent by an attorney must be used for the benefit of the donor, *not* the attorney.

Where to Look for Power of Attorney Documents

Since the power of attorney documents are not usually given in advance to the representative who will exercise them, the documents may be stored in several places. If the location of someone's power of attorney documents is not known, the next of kin or representative should search for the documents in these places:

- Lawyer's office: the patient may have left a copy at the lawyer's office along with a will.
- Safety deposit box in a financial institution
- Safe or lock-box at home
- Personal papers filing cabinet at home

Once the power of attorney documents have been located, the holders of the power can then present the power of attorney document, along with personal identification, to banks or other institutions in order to take care of the disabled person's financial, legal, property and cash flow affairs. (Usually, the lawyer will have made several notarized copies for the donor in advance, or can make some for the attorneys when they must act.)

Using the Power of Attorney for Property on Behalf of the Person With a Disability

Janet's story

Every hospital I was in asked for power of attorney—but didn't specify Power of Attorney for Personal Care! When Marie and Gavin tried to handle my bank accounts by presenting the power of attorney (for Property) to the banks in question, the first question asked was, "Can we talk to Ms. Freedman to verify this?" The answer, of course, was "No, she is in intensive care on a ventilator and cannot speak! That is why we have the power of attorney!"

Once the power of attorney document has been located, the holders of the power can then present the power of attorney document, along with personal identification, to banks or other institutions in order to take care of the disabled person's financial, legal, property and cash flow affairs.

But be warned! Many front-line staff in financial institutions do not understand what a power of attorney is and how it can be used by the donor's legal representative. Most often, the front-line staff will enquire if the holders have one of the institution's own power of attorney documents signed by the donor. In most cases, the answer will be "no." Some financial institution staff then conclude that the general power of attorney presented is suspect or invalid. The next question from the staff member may be whether they can contact the donor for verification! If the donor were able to verify the power of attorney, the chances are they would not require the services of the legal representative acting on their behalf! The general, enduring or continuing power of attorney is valid in all institutions: it's the staff who have not been trained to appreciate that fact.

It is not uncommon for the representatives to have to contact a senior officer in a bank or trust company in order to deal with the donor's accounts.

Who Needs to Know About Someone's Disability?

When a disability occurs, several people must be notified.

Immediate notification:
- Police (If an accident has occurred, this happens automatically)
- Spouse
- Children
- Personal representative (holder of power of attorney, holder of Directive for Personal Care;)
- Workplace, business associates

The patient's parents should be notified, depending on their circumstances. The shock may be too great and delay may be wise.

Secondary notification:

- Other close relatives
- Friends
- Business associates not directly associated with the patient
- Clients (if self-employed)

Importance of Communication

The holders of the power of attorney need to be kept informed of the patient's situation once the power of attorney is exercised. Although the family will be informed directly of the patient's situation, the attorneys may have difficulty in getting information.

The details on the patient's condition are important to the attorneys for these reasons:

- The attorneys are responsible for the patient/donor's financial situation. They need to know if the patient will require assistive devices and private care after release from hospital. They must arrange funding for such services or devices.
- The attorneys may need to apply to government agencies, such as Canada Pension Plan, to obtain disability benefits for the patient. All medical details must be entered on the form.
- The attorneys must notify the patient's disability insurance company of the patient's situation and initiate the claim for benefits. The forms require medical data which the attorneys must obtain.
- The physicians' estimates of how long it will be before the patient returns to work are important to the attorneys for planning purposes. As an example, patients who have small businesses may not require certain services—such as office space—which can be disposed of by the attorneys to save money.
- If the patient's medical prognosis is bleak, and prospects for earning income in the foreseeable future are slight, the attorneys may have to

consider the sale of assets such as cars or even the home. It is important that the attorneys be kept up to date on all details of the patient's progress. Obviously, the attorneys would prefer to keep as many assets intact as possible. But if the patient's debts cannot be paid in any other way, then assets must be sold to meet these obligations.

- In some instances, after evaluation by rehabilitation specialists, it may be decided that the patient's home cannot be modified to allow him or her safety and mobility upon release from hospital. In such cases, selling the home and moving the patient to a new type of residence may the solution. The attorneys must act in such cases to get the best possible price for the existing home while finding a more suitable residence at an affordable price.
- The holders of the power of attorney must keep records of the financial transactions they undertake on behalf of the donor/patient. The attorneys can be held legally responsible for actions and decisions they take during the time they exercised power of attorney for the donor, if these actions were contrary to the best interests of the donor/patient. This liability can extend beyond the donor to the beneficiaries of the donor's estate — this means that the attorney has a responsibility not just to the donor but to the beneficiaries of the donor's estate if the donor were to die.

Record Keeping

The attorneys need to keep such records as:
- Net worth of donor at the time the attorneys assumed control
- Cash flow (money coming in as income and going out as expenses) from the time the attorneys assumed control

- Updated bank statements and bank books
- Details of investment income received
- Up-to-date statements on RRSP's
- Copies of latest income tax returns and any dealings with Canada Customs and Revenue Agency (CCRA), including Assessment forms.
- Records of the donor's business income and expenses (if the attorneys are empowered to act concerning the business)
- Copies of invoices received and paid

Provincial Legislation

In most provinces, the strength behind a power of attorney comes from a combination of legislation, often a Powers of Attorney Act and another statute relating to property ownership. In Ontario and British Columbia, the *enduring* aspect of a power of attorney is provided by a third piece of legislation: the Substitute Decisions Act in Ontario and the Representation Agreement Act in British Columbia. In these two provinces, the Powers of Attorney Acts now deal exclusively with property or financial matters, and more specifically, only powers of attorney that do not survive the incapacity of the donor. In other words, these acts are not used for continuing or enduring powers of attorney, which is covered under the Substitute Decisions Act or the Representation Agreement Acts in Ontario and British Columbia, respectively. Find a lawyer who works in the area of trusts and estates, including powers of attorney, through your provincial Law Society office.

A Note About Mandates in the Province of Quebec

Although Québec is governed by the Civil Code, instead of Common Law, a *mandate given in anticipation of incapacity* under the Civil Code operates with a similar effect. In fact, the document describing the mandate is referred to as a power of attorney. A mandate may be given for property and financial matters and/or health care matters.

The mandate under the Quebec Civil Code assumes that only simple administrative powers are being given, that is, that the holder of the mandate can perform only those tasks necessary to preserve the individual's property, such as making mortgage and utility payments, administering bank accounts and preparing income tax returns.

Full administrative powers would allow the holder to sell property without the approval of the courts. This can be set up specifically within the mandate. One document can cover personal care, finances, and "living will" directives in one document. The *mandatary* (person to whom power is given on behalf of the donor, known as the *mandator*), must apply to the courts to certify incapacity before it comes into effect.

A note about Henson Trusts

See Chapter 8, "Provincial Government Benefits" for a full discussion of using Henson trusts to look after the interests of adult disabled children in the event of the deaths of their parents.

POWER OF ATTORNEY FOR PERSONAL CARE

The second form of power of attorney is called a *Power of Attorney for Personal Care*, and is sometimes referred to as a *Living Will*. In British Columbia, the Representative Agreement Act allows for the writing of a Living Will. In Ontario, the Substitute Decisions Act provides for Power of Attorney for Personal Care and allows a person to set up a Living Will document. A Living Will or Power of Attorney for Personal Care or Advanced Directive is a document in which you, as the donor of the power of attorney, allow the attorney to make decisions about your health care treatment. It can be set up without a lawyer's input, but it is advisable to have a lawyer review the provisions of the document to ensure that they are enforceable.

Some people think that without the Power of Attorney for Personal Care, nobody will be able to make those important decisions on their behalf. This is not true. Medical professionals will always try to obtain consent for any treatment decisions from the patient first and then from the next of kin. If the people you would name are in fact your next of kin, then a Power of Attorney for Personal Care may not be necessary.

All provinces recognize Living Wills, except for the province of New Brunswick. There is also no provision for Living Wills in the Territories. This is a grey area of the law at present. The Attorney for Personal Care may be asked to decide on life and death matters: should extraordinary measures be taken to keep the patient alive? Will attending physicians follow the measures laid out in the Personal Care Power of Attorney or Advance Care Directive? (Some may not if they fear legal repercussions from the next of kin.) Should certain experimental procedures or medications be administered to the patient whose chances of survival or recovery may be lessened without such attempts? Some people do not wish to put such directives in a document that may have to be used in uncertain circumstances in the future. They would rather their next of kin make decisions, if and when, certain possibilities occur in the course of hospitalization or care.

If no Power of Attorney for Personal Care exists, then the next of kin will be asked to give instructions. But it is advisable for individuals who intend to give Power of Attorney for Personal Care to have these instructions set up in a legal format.

Assuming you have set up power of attorney documents for both Personal Care and Legal and Property affairs, your next of kin must find the actual documents that give these powers.

Sarah's story

> *Sarah, a single person in her forties, was injured in a vicious assault. During her recuperation, her Attorney for Property was besieged by several of Sarah's well-meaning friends as to how matters should have been handled. In addition, several friends tried to intervene in matters of Sarah's care. Had Sarah set up a Power of Attorney for Personal Care with named attorneys, the health care practitioners would have followed the instructions of one attorney, and not been concerned with the opinions of those who were not empowered as Sarah's attorneys.*

Legislation Governing Power of Attorney for Personal Care and Living Wills

For those provinces that do recognize living wills, the scope and relevant legislation is summarized in Table 2, below. Some provinces recognize only *proxy directives* and others recognize both *proxy* and *instructional directives*. A proxy directive is one that gives powers to someone else to make decisions on your behalf; an instructional directive is where the instructions for personal care are actually written into the document itself. These tables are provided as an overview only, to illustrate the complexity and diversity between the provinces. If you wish to learn more about a particular province's legislation, we recommend that you obtain a copy of the legislation from that province's official publications office.

Table 1
Provincial Legislation Relevant to the Power of Attorney for Property

Alberta	Powers of Attorney Act (includes reference to the Enduring Power of Attorney)
	Land Titles Act
British Columbia	Representation Agreement Act
	Power of Attorney Act
	Land Title Act
Manitoba	The Powers of Attorney Act
	The Mental Health Act
	The Homesteads Act
	The Real Property Act
New Brunswick	Property Act
Newfoundland & Labrador	Enduring Powers of Attorney Act
	Registration of Deeds Act
Nova Scotia	Powers of Attorney Act
	Registry Act
Ontario	Substitute Decisions Act, as modified by the Advocacy, Consent and Substitution Decisions Statute Law Amendment Act (Bill 19)
	Land Titles Act/ Family Law Act
	Registry Act
	Powers of Attorney Act
Prince Edward Island	Powers of Attorney Act
	Land Titles Act
Québec	Civil Code, Book 5, Title 2, Chapter 9
Saskatchewan	The Powers of Attorney Act
	The Homesteads Act
	The Land Titles Act

Table 2
Summary of Provincial Living Will Legislation

Province	Legislation	Scope
Alberta	The Personal Directives Act S.A.1996, as amended, 1997.	• Recognizes both proxy and instructional directives. • Allows the maker or donor to provide "advance personal instructions regarding their own personal matters while recognizing that such instructions cannot include instructions related to aided suicide, euthanasia or other instructions prohibited by law". • A personal directive, or part of a personal directive, only comes into effect with respect to a personal matter when the donor lacks capacity with respect to that matter.
British Columbia	The Representation Agreement Act R.S.B.C. 1996, as amended, 1999. This act covers both powers of attorney for property and living wills.	• Recognizes proxy and instructional directives • May specify what types of decisions the representative (holder) can make on behalf of the donor. • If the representation agreement grants the representative *exceptional powers*, then the donor must consult with a lawyer. Exceptional powers include, for example, the representative's right to give consent for treatment under certain

Province	Legislation	Scope
		circumstances even if the donor is refusing to give consent for that treatment. • A representation agreement comes into force as soon as it is registered, unless the agreement specifically states that it is only to come into effect at a certain time or when a triggering event occurs.
Manitoba	The Health Care Directives Act C.C.S.M.1992.	• Recognizes both proxy and instructional directives. • Can give instructions regarding any health care decisions that the donor would be allowed to make if mentally capable. Cannot include instructions related to non-beneficial treatment or aided suicide. • A health care directive comes into effect when the donor ceases to have the capacity to make a decision regarding a proposed treatment.
New Brunswick	Not applicable	• N/A
Newfoundland & Labrador	The Advance Health Care Directives Act R.S.N.1995.	• Recognizes both proxy and instructional directives dealing with personal health care. • May contain instructions that the donor is not to receive certain medical treatment (including life-prolonging treatment) in specified circumstances. However, instructions

Province	Legislation	Scope
		that would, if followed, amount to euthanasia will not be effective. • An advance health care directive comes into effect when the donor no longer has the capacity to make health care decisions.
Nova Scotia	Medical Consent Act, R.S.N.S.1989.	• This Act does not expressly deal with living wills or powers of attorney. However, Section 2 of the Act allows an individual who is capable of giving consent or directions regarding medical treatment to authorize another person to give that consent at those times when he/she is unable to do so. While this amounts to a proxy directive, there is no provision to give binding directions to the chosen representative (holder). (Although guidelines can be included, the representative may not be legally bound to follow them.)
Ontario	Substitute Decisions Act (SDA), 1992, as amended, 1998 and the Health Care and Consent Act (HCCA), 1996 as amended 2000	• Part II of the Substitute Decisions Act allows an individual to appoint a substitute decision maker (i.e., attorney, holder) to make health care decisions on his/her behalf if he/she becomes incapable of making those decisions him/herself.

Province	Legislation	Scope
		• The Health Care and Consent Act (HCCA) allows the donor to give his/her attorney binding instructions regarding the refusal of or consent to medical treatment in specified circumstances. *Treatment* refers to virtually anything done for medical or health-related reasons.
		• A Power of Attorney for Personal Care comes into effect if the HCCA applies to the decision and the Act authorizes the attorney to make that decision or, if the HCCA does not apply to that decision, if the attorney has reasonable grounds to believe the maker is incapable of making the decision. The latter may be subject to a condition requiring the confirmation of the maker's incapacity.
Prince Edward Island	The Consent to Treatment and Health Care S.P.E.I 2000	• Recognizes both proxy and instructional directives.
		• If an individual fails to appoint a proxy and then becomes incapable of making his/her own decisions, then the following persons will be entitled to make those decisions on his/her behalf, in preferential order: guardian with authority; spouse; son, daughter, parent or person with parental

Province	Legislation	Scope
		authority; brother or sister; known trusted friend; any other relative.
		• The authority of a proxy comes into effect when the donor ceases to be capable of making or communicating decisions, or upon some other triggering event specified in the directive.
Quebec	Civil Code of Lower Canada, S.Q. 1991 Quebec Civil Code as amended, 1999	• In Quebec, individuals can execute a "mandate given in anticipation of incapacity" for either property or personal care. This differs from a proxy in that it survives the incapacity of the maker, while a proxy executed in Quebec does not. The appointed substitute decision maker is called the *mandatary*.
		• The mandate only comes into effect when the donor (called the *mandator*) becomes incapable.
		• A mandate for the protection of the donor can contain specific instructions regarding the refusal of or consent to treatment, or it can contain general principles to guide the mandatary.
Saskatchewan	The Health Care Directives and Substitute Health Care Decision Makers Act S.S.1997.	• Recognizes both proxy and instructional directives.
		• Part II - If an individual fails to appoint a proxy and he/she becomes

Province	Legislation	Scope
		incapable of making his/her own decisions, then the nearest relative will be entitled to make those decisions on his/her behalf. The nearest relative is the first person on the following list who is willing, available and has the capacity to make the health care decision: spouse or common-law spouse, adult son or daughter, parent or legal custodian, adult brother or sister, grandparent, adult grandchild, adult aunt or uncle, adult nephew or niece.
		• The authority of a proxy comes into effect when the donor does not have the capacity to make a health care decision regarding a proposed treatment.

SOURCES OF INFORMATION

<u>The Canadian Guide to Will and Estate Planning</u>, by Douglas Gray and John Budd. 2nd edition. McGraw-Hill Ryerson, 2002.

<u>The Estate Planner's Handbook</u>, by Robert Spenceley. CCH, 2002.

<u>You Can't Take It With You, by Sandra Foster</u>. 4th edition. John Wiley and Sons, 2002.

<u>How to Inherit Money</u>, by Michael Alexander. Harper Business, 1997.

Provincial Law Societies have guides to selecting lawyers and often provide taped telephone information on various legal topics. They have lists of lawyers with their specialties noted.

Check your *provincial government Web site* (see *Resources* section at back of this book for Web sites) for "Ministry of the Attorney General" for information on power of attorney, living wills, trusteeship, guardianship and wills. Or look in your telephone directory under government listings.

GLOSSARY

Attorney: Person who acts on behalf of another person, through a power of attorney document, in property, financial, or legal matters; or for personal care.
The individual acts on behalf of the other person when the individual granting or donating the power is incapacitated. However, the individual who acts for another person is not usually an attorney in the sense of a lawyer.

Alternate Attorney: Someone who is named by the donor to step in to replace the originally appointed attorney if that person is unable to fulfill his/her responsibilities as attorney.

Donor: Person who gives the power, the right and the responsibility to act on his/her behalf, (in legal, financial or property matters, or for personal care), to another person, through a power of attorney document,.

Fiduciary: Individuals or an institution which is legally obligated to act on behalf of another party or person. The duty of a fiduciary is at the highest level of care. They must act ethically on behalf of the other individual on financial, legal and property matters. Failure to do so can result in charges of fraud against the fiduciary (who may be called an attorney, executor or trustee).

Instructional Directive: A legal document giving someone authority to act on behalf of another person with regard to personal care. The instructions for personal care which the donor wishes the donee to follow are written into this document.

Mandate: Under the Quebec Civil Code, the equivalent of power of attorney in the Common Law provinces.

Mandator: Under the Quebec Civil Code, the equivalent of donor in the Common Law provinces.

Mandatary: Under the Quebec Civil Code, the equivalent of attorney (person who holds the power to act from the mandatory to act on the mandator's behalf).

Proxy: A legal document which authorizes another party to act for someone else in legal, financial or property matters; also, the individual who acts on someone else's behalf.

Proxy directive: A legal document which authorizes another person to act for someone else by making healthcare decisions on the donor's behalf.

Triggering event: The starting point from which the holder of a power of attorney may begin to act on behalf of the donor who grants or donates the power. The event may be the donor's mental or physical incapacity as determined by a qualified medical practitioner. If no triggering event is stipulated in the power of attorney document, then the attorney has the power to act from the time the document is signed.

CHAPTER 4

DISABILITY INSURANCE

Marie's story

The first question Janet's associates asked after calling to find out how she was progressing was this: "Does she have enough disability insurance?" Yes, as a good financial planner, Janet did take out disability insurance—as much as she was able—but there is never "enough" coverage when a disability strikes.

Most people know how life insurance works: someone dies, the insurance company pays out a benefit to the survivors to replace the breadwinner's or insured person's current income and potential future income. What about situations in which the person doesn't die: they are alive, but unable to work? This is when disability insurance is needed.

Disability insurance is really income-replacement insurance. The money that the policy pays replaces a portion of the income that would normally have come into the household if the person with the disability had been working.

Most individuals employed full-time in large corporations and public sector organizations have a disability plan as part of their benefits. There is usually a Short-Term Accident and Sickness program that begins at the start of an illness or disability.

After a certain number of weeks, Long Term Disability (LTD) Plan benefits begin. Even these employer-sponsored LTD programs, however, may have *maximum dollar payout* provisions, for example, no more than $2,000 per month paid out in benefits. This means that higher income employees may not receive enough to maintain their living standards. In some situations, these policies can be added to, or *topped up*, by privately paid policies.

The main sources of disability income insurance are as follows:

- Group disability plans through employers
- Professional group plans offered by professional associations (engineers, doctors, lawyers, etc.)
- Group disability plans such as university alumni associations
- Affinity group plans as offered by Boards of Trade and Chambers of Commerce, etc. (The cost is modest for the basic coverage usually offered.) Membership in the Board or Chamber is required to join these plans.
- Federal Government through the Canada Pension Plan (See Chapter 7, "Federal Government Programs.")
- Private disability plans bought by individuals, particularly those who are small business owners, entrepreneurs or consultants.

Disability insurance is costly if you must pay for it yourself, whereas group plans are relatively inexpensive for employees to purchase. It's worthwhile, however, to keep the cost in context. How much do you pay monthly for car insurance—hoping it will not be needed, but knowing that it is essential for your financial and legal well-being? In Canada's largest cities, even with a top-rated auto policy, you are probably paying at least $100 per month in premiums. For the same amount, a 40-year old non-smoker could probably get disability insurance that would pay over $1,000 per month in the event of a disability.

Disability insurance is sold by agents licensed by life insurance companies to sell disability insurance. General insurance agents, who are licensed to sell only home and auto insurance, do not sell disability insurance, although they may sell out-of-country medical insurance.

In this chapter, the focus is on the general principles of disability insurance, especially privately purchased policies.

DETERMINING THE COST OF DISABILITY INSURANCE

As with all insurance, disability insurance carriers set up criteria for coverage: who will be covered, under what conditions and at what price. They must balance the *risk* of offering the insurance against the expected *return on investment* to the company from premiums and investment income. Insurance companies make their money by investing your premiums in the stock, bond, and real estate markets. They also consider the *claims experience* of the past. In other words, they ask how likely it is that a certain category of policyholder will claim on their policies based on their past experience with other policyholders.

Underwriting Factors

Insurance companies first of all determine which categories of individuals they will cover. The risk factors that insurance companies consider in issuing policies are as follows:
- Occupation
- Lifestyle
- Age
- Sex
- Health
- Income

Occupation
How likely is it that the person in a broad class of employment will become injured on the job or suffer a type of disability for which the insurance company must pay out under the policy? The past claims experience determines how a particular occupation will be rated.

Someone who works at a desk all day is not at as high risk as a person who works in construction, for example. Some occupational groups can purchase only limited disability coverage, whereas others can obtain enhanced benefits coverage. Some workers may not be insurable at all under disability policies because their occupations are too risky (i.e., the probability of claims is too high).

Furthermore, what may be a disabling injury in one occupation may not be so in another. A broken leg doesn't interfere with a computer operator's ability to work, but it would mean that a truck driver could not perform his or her work; thus, it is a disability that prevents a person from earning a living. Some occupations are seasonal in nature, and this also affects the insurance rating on those occupations.

Lifestyle

Risky behaviour or *high-risk lifestyle* activities, such as piloting a small plane or bungee jumping, or even horseback riding, usually results in exclusions in the policy for these types of activities. This means if you are injured while doing any of these activities, your policy will not cover you.

Age

The older you are, the more likely it is that you are going to have a claim, and therefore, the higher the premium cost. You can apply for disability insurance as an individual up to age 59 or 60, depending on the policy and the company. The benefit period can go to age 65 or beyond if you purchase *lifetime accident,* or *sickness* as an *optional rider.*

Sex

Women live longer than men, and that is why life insurance costs less for women than men. Women pay more for disability insurance than their male counterparts because of increased *morbidity.* Morbidity means the likelihood of developing a disease or other health impairment. In other words, women tend to develop more disabilities before age 65 than men do.

Health

When you apply for disability insurance, you are asked to disclose all relevant or material information about your health. The application is very detailed, especially in the area of health history and family medical history. Certain health factors may mean that you may be more likely to make a claim than someone without such health concerns. Insurance companies consider these factors when they underwrite an insurance policy.

Some *pre-existing conditions* may prevent a person from obtaining disability coverage. The questionnaires that insurance companies make you complete usually include requests for detailed reports from family physicians as well as a medical examination by a nurse who works on behalf of the insurance company. Depending on which pre-existing conditions are brought to light in these questionnaires and medical statements, you may or may not get coverage by the insurance company. These conditions may be such things as a family medical history of heart disease, cancer, treatment for stress and depression, and lifestyle issues. Currently, since treatment for stress and depression has increased significantly, many insurance companies will not cover people with a history of these treatments. In many cases, the insurance company may issue the policy with an exclusion rider that rules out the specific pre-existing condition. This means that the policy will cover you only for those disabilities not related to your pre-existing condition. This is a common practice in the area of stress. The insurance company will apply a *nervous mental disorder exclusion* to the policy, which can be removed at a later date if the cause of the stress no longer exists.

Applicants for disability insurance must respond to all questions honestly. If, in the event of a claim, the insurance company can prove that you withheld information or deliberately misled the insurance company in any way about pre-existing conditions, then the claim may be denied.

Income

Your application for disability insurance will also ask questions about your income. Disability insurance is intended to replace only a percentage of normal income earned before a disability—usually between 66.6% and 80% of gross prior income. This percentage may be higher in the lower tax brackets and lower in the higher tax brackets to reflect the differences in tax rates. The goal of the insurance company is to get the person with the disability back to work. So the benefits paid are less than what claimants would earn if they were at work, as an incentive to get back to work—if it is possible to do so.

With many disability insurance plans, the coverage paid by the insurance company is often *integrated with* (reduced by) the amount of payment received from other sources. Such sources include workers' compensation benefits, Canada Pension Plan (CPP) disability benefits or payouts from an insurance claim in the event of a car accident, to name a few.

Generally speaking, it is not possible to replace 100% of a person's pre-disability income through disability insurance policies, except through some professional association group plans and individual policies. These may cover up to 100% of income in certain circumstances. The main reason for this is that employer group plans *offset* for CPP or other disability benefits. This means that the total of all disability claims payments from all insurance companies cannot add up to more than 85% of the individual's pre-disability income.

Some group insurance plans provide a base level of $1,000 monthly income that is reduced by any CPP disability income received. This type of policy really provides virtually nothing to the person with a serious disability. For example, someone who has been earning at least $40,000 for several years could expect to receive a disability income of about $960 per month from the CPP disability plan if they qualified under CPP rules. In this instance, the disability insurance would only pay $40 per month ($1,000 - $960) to the person with the disability.

An individual policy that you pay for privately will not normally integrate with CPP, but it may well integrate with other group or individual disability coverage.

Policy Definitions

The more specific the definitions are in a disability contract, the more clarity there is in terms of the obligations of both parties. How much "wiggle room" is there in the contract? With some contracts, the *policyholder* (i.e., the insured person) wants and receives maximum flexibility. In others, the insurance company has a tight set of obligations to which the company is committed and that prevents the policyholder from receiving expanded benefits. But the definitions in the policy have a price. The more broadly the contract can be construed to be in favour of you, the policyholder, the higher your cost in the form of premiums for the duration and type of benefits to be received. In other words, the better the plan from the policyholder's point of view, the higher the cost of the premiums.

Key definitions in a disability policy contract are as follows:

- The definition of disability
- Occupational definitions
- Duration of coverage
- Definitions related to the policy's *continuance*, which refers to when the policy is *in force*, for

example, the conditions under which it can be cancelled or renewed.

Disability definitions

All disability insurance contracts give a definition of both *total disability* and *partial disability.*

Total disability, in most contracts, means a condition that meets *all* of the following requirements:

- The condition is due to injury or sickness, and
- The applicant receives the regular care and attendance of a doctor appropriate for the condition, or the condition is such that the regular care and attendance of a doctor is unlikely to result in any improvement in the condition, and
- The condition results in a loss of earned income of 75% or more, or it results in the applicant being unable to perform the important duties of his or her *regular occupation,* and the applicant is not engaged in any other occupation.

Partial disability means:

- That the applicant is not totally disabled, but
- The applicant is unable to perform one or more of the important duties of his or her occupation, or
- The applicant is unable to work at least 50% of the time.

Residual disability means:

- That the applicant is not totally disabled, but
- As a result of disability, the applicant is experiencing a loss of income of at least 20%, but less than 75%, of normal income.

Occupational definitions

The definition of what constitutes the policyholder's occupation is critical. It determines whether the policyholder can obtain and maintain benefits over a period of time or whether the policyholder must accept employment that he or she would not have considered before the disability.

Below are the standard definitions of occupation typically found in disability insurance contracts, both group and privately owned:

Own Occupation: This is the best insurance definition, usually reserved for professionals and very high-income earners who are eligible for the top insurance classification. It is usually purchased as an option on individual plans and it is expensive. Your *own occupation* is the job you were doing just prior to the disability. It means that, as long as you cannot perform the duties of your *own* occupation, even if you return to work in a *different* occupation, you will still be considered disabled and will be paid full benefits *regardless* of what you are earning in your new occupation. Take the example of the medical surgeon who loses fingers and cannot return to surgery, but can teach. In this circumstance, the disability income would be paid in full each month even though he or she has a different job that pays well (or more in some cases).

Regular occupation: This definition refers to the job that you did just prior to the disability. You will be considered disabled if you are unable to perform the duties of your occupation *and are not working in another occupation. Regular occupation* coverage can cover you for 1 or 2 years, 5 years or as long as the benefit period runs, for example, to age 65, depending on the policy terms. This definition is found in most insurance plans, both group and individual.

The key question here is how long are you protected in your regular occupation? If it is an employer group plan, the contract may state 1 or 2 years. In that case, after the 1 or 2 years are up, you would be expected to take other work if you were able. This other work does not mean you have to sell pencils on the street, and you cannot be forced to accept employment that is not consistent with your training, education, and experience.

Any Occupation by virtue of training, education, and experience: This definition means that you must take another occupation if you are able to work in a field for which you were previously trained, in which you had previous experience, or for which you have the necessary educational qualifications. This requirement normally follows on from a period of time of 1 or 2 to 5 years of regular occupation coverage and is fairly typical for most group policies. Most group policies have the regular occupation definition followed by *any occupation by virtue of training, education, and experience.*

Any occupation: This definition means that you must be unable to work at any job. Traditionally, this definition is rarely seen. But it is important for consumers to be aware of this definition, especially since there are now concerns that, with claims levels rising, insurance companies may require a pure *any occupation* definition after 2 years in some group plans. The problem with an *any occupation* definition is that you have to be unable to do anything— telemarketing or selling pencils on the street— regardless of your previous occupation, education, or training.

✘ Warning: Due to ever-increasing disability insurance claims, some group policy definitions are likely to require an *any occupation by virtue of education, training, or experience* immediately rather than allowing 1 or 2 years of coverage while you cannot perform your *regular occupation* first. This trend means that you must be alert to occupational definitions. Many people may have to purchase individual coverage as a top-up where appropriate.

Duration of Coverage

It is not uncommon for people to suffer lingering effects from their disability for a prolonged period of time, to the extent that they are unable to perform the duties of their regular or own occupation. However, they can do some limited forms of work. Sometimes there is pressure on the policyholder from the insurance company to retrain in a new occupation. If the individual refuses to retrain, then it is likely that the insurance company will stop the benefits.

Some points for consideration:

- In shopping for a disability policy, most people should select a policy with a *regular occupation* definition as a minimum.
- The duration of regular occupation coverage in a privately purchased disability plan can go beyond the normal 2-year or 5-year terms and can go to age 65 (or older if negotiated). A policy with regular occupation coverage for 2 to 5 years should be the absolute minimum. The policy should revert to the *any occupation by virtue of training education and experience* after the term of regular occupation coverage expires.
- A plan with *any occupation* coverage should not be purchased.
- If you are close to age 60, you should consider whether it is worthwhile to choose a plan that will cover you under *regular occupation* for a 5-year term instead of one that covers you until age 65. For example, a 58-year-old would have lower premiums by selecting a 5-year plan than a plan with coverage to age 65. Would the extra 3 years of coverage to age 65 be worth the additional cost? However, for people in their thirties or forties, it would be worthwhile to pay the extra premiums to ensure adequate coverage.
- Do you enjoy your current occupation? If you are ambivalent, or would welcome retraining, then

regular occupation coverage is not as crucial and a policy of any occupation by virtue of training, education and experience coverage may be more appropriate. In the event of disability, you could be re-trained for something that may be of more interest to you.

Policy Continuance Definitions

Under what conditions will the disability insurance policy continue in force under the contract as signed? You want to maintain coverage that is most beneficial to you; the insurance company may decide after a period of claims experience that policies need to be modified. But modifications to existing policies may not meet with your approval. You entered into a contract in good faith. Therefore, insurance companies offer certain guarantees (at increased cost), to policyholders to maintain certain features. Without these guarantees, the insurance company can make premium changes to, or even cancel, policies.

There are three types of policy continuance features:
- Guaranteed Renewable and Non-cancellable
- Guaranteed Renewable
- Cancellable/Renewable at the option of the insurance company

Guaranteed Renewable and Non-cancellable policies

Guaranteed renewable and non-cancellable policies give you the right to renew the policy to a specified age (typically no older than between ages 65 to 75), regardless of any changes in health or occupation. The premium remains the same to age 65 and thereafter is based on your continuing to work full-time. The premiums are at the prevailing rate at that time. In the event of a claim, benefits are normally only payable for 2 years after age 65.

Guaranteed renewable

A *guaranteed renewable* policy allows the insurance company to make future premium changes for all policyholders within a class if the insurance company detects a negative trend over time. The premium increase cannot be applied to one policyholder in the class, but must be applied to all members of the class.

Cancellable policies

With *cancellable policies*, the insurance company can change the premiums or cancel or not renew the policy for a class of policyholders altogether if claims experience deteriorates. This type of policy is being used more and more to cover people who would not otherwise be eligible for coverage. Examples are people in high-risk occupations, part-time workers, newly self-employed people, some home-based workers, and those with low income. Insurance companies may permit these policyholders to transfer to more traditional disability policies at a later date subject to medical examination.

Policy Options, Riders and Exclusions

Waiting period or elimination period

The period of time between the start of the disability and the start of benefit payments is the *waiting period* or the *elimination period*. The longer this waiting period, the lower the premium cost. In some cases, due to good luck or good medical care, many people are able to recover during the waiting period and never need to collect on their disability policies.

Group disability insurance plans normally have a waiting period of 26 weeks. This is because the employee with a disability will be receiving payments from group short-term sickness/illness/accident plans or from accumulated sick leave and then from Employment Insurance (EI) benefits for 15 weeks (after a 2-week waiting period).

Individuals with privately held plans have to decide when they want benefits to start. The length of the elimination period is one of the major components of the disability premium. You, the policyholder, have to consider these facts:

- If you are self-employed or run a small business, you are not going to receive EI benefits; therefore, there is no 15-week cushion of income.
- Do you have other income streams available to cover short-term disability? Someone who has followed the principles of financial planning and has set aside, or has easy access to, 3 months of living expenses, will not need to start disability insurance for at least 3 months after the onset of disability.
- A business person, who always has at least 3 months receivables in hand, may also not need to start coverage until that period is over.
- Someone for whom money is always tight will need to have some insurance starting quite soon after the start of the disability. In this case, you need to make sure that your benefits start after a shorter waiting period, for example 30 days.
- One way to reduce costs is to split start dates for different portions of the policy over several months.

Janet's story

I had coverage of $2,000 per month starting over a period of 6 months. Three hundred dollars kicked in after 30 days; another $600 started after 90 days; the next $1000 started after 120 days and the balance after 180 days. Having a staggered approach helped enormously—since I spent 5 months in the hospital, my expenses during that time were very basic. The full amount of coverage therefore started as I returned home.

Partial disability provisions

What happens if you are able to start working again, but only part-time, whether 2 hours a day or 2 days a week? Insurance companies address this with two different types of partial disability provisions:

Standard partial disability coverage

Each insurance company, and even each policy, may have a different definition of what constitutes partial disability, and for how long benefits will be paid. For example, Policy A may provide a partial disability benefit of 50% of the total coverage for a period of 6 months.

Policy B may provide partial disability benefits up to 75% for the first 3 months; 50% for the next 3 months and a declining amount thereafter for an additional 6 months. Policy C may offer 24 months of partial disability benefits: 50% for 12 months and 25% for 12 months.

The costs for these three different options will also be different with option A being the least expensive and option C the most expensive.

Residual income loss replacement coverage

Residual income loss replacement coverage is top-of-the-line coverage for partial disability, usually found only in policies for executives and self-employed professionals. Ongoing partial disability can be covered until age 65 or to the end of the term of the policy, with adjustments made on a monthly basis according to how much net business income loss there has been in that month. For example, if a self-employed person's pre-disability net income (gross income less business expenses) was $4,000 per month and they have coverage for $2,000 per month, then net business earnings of $1,000 per month (25% of the pre-disability income) during this residual period would reduce the disability payment by 25% or $500 per month. (See Chapter 10, "Disability and the Self-employed Small Business Person.")

Consider the value of these different options according to a particular person's circumstances. Someone who is younger and has many more years of working life ahead of them is best advised to take residual income loss coverage over partial disability benefits. An older professional or self-employed person, though, may not consider that the extra premium is worthwhile. Residual income benefits are significantly more expensive than partial coverage, simply because they can potentially pay out for a much longer period of time. Of course, some policies may offer residual income benefits for a short period of time. Fewer and fewer companies are offering residual income benefits. Some insurance companies offer the choice of either a residual income benefit or partial disability benefit option to be chosen at the time a disability claim is made. There are options for partial disability benefits, payable over different time frames at different percentages, again to be selected at the time of a claim.

Rehabilitation Benefits

Some policies include rehabilitation benefits as part of the package. What is defined as a rehabilitation benefit varies from insurance company to insurance company and from policy to policy. Typically, rehabilitation benefits include such therapies as physiotherapy, occupational therapy, or psychological counselling that assist the patient in returning to work and in maintaining optimum working capacity. It can also include computer upgrades, voice recognition software, and any other equipment to enable the person with the disability to return to the workforce as quickly as possible.

Usually, in these situations, the insurance company hires a rehabilitation consultant who assesses and assists the person with the disability to obtain the most useful equipment and therapies for his/her situation.

Waiver of Premiums

While you collect disability insurance, the premium cost of the disability policy is waived (stopped). The premium waiver may begin at the *onset* of disability, or in most cases, after you have been disabled for 3 months or on claim for 3 months. This option is normally included in the policy at no extra cost.

Cost of Living Adjustment

The cost of living adjustment or COLA is the inflation-protection rider on the disability policy.

During the 1970s and 1980s, when inflation was rampant, individual disability policies almost always included *Cost of Living Adjustment* (COLA) clauses. During the 1990s, as inflation rates declined worldwide, COLA clauses fell out of favour. Since all extra benefits or riders have a price tag attached, they were often omitted from individual policies.

All COLA clauses state a maximum amount of inflationary increase that the policy will pay in any one year, usually around 4% to 5% per year. In some cases—and at a significant cost—policies will pay up to 10%. Although the Bank of Canada is insisting that we are unlikely to see the rampant inflation of the 1970s and 1980s again, the reality is that increases in heating costs, gasoline prices and other everyday expenses can have a significant impact on income needs, especially for those living on fixed incomes. In a worst-case scenario, a person with a disability could be collecting disability insurance for 30 years or more, which is where the benefit of COLA is obvious. In some cases, when the policy includes residual income loss coverage, not only are the benefits indexed to inflation, but also the pre-disability income levels are adjusted upwards by the same amount. Even at a modest inflation rate, income needs can double over a period of 30 years.

Right to Purchase Additional Coverage (Future Insurability Option)

Some privately purchased policies include an option to purchase additional coverage of up to 100% of the original face value over time without the policyholder having to undergo another medical. There is an additional premium for this option.

Janet's story

When I took out disability insurance coverage almost 20 years ago, the original benefit amount was $1,000 per month. Over time, I took advantage of the option to increase coverage to $2,000 without having to undergo medicals. The premium on the additional coverage was higher, though, to reflect my increasing age.

Return of Premiums Option

Disability insurance is *pure* insurance: it does not normally have any investment component built into it. However, some insurance companies do offer a type of investment return, but once again, there is a price!

Usually the cost for a *return of premiums option* is an additional 50% of the cost of the premium each year. For example, if the annual premium is $1,000, the *return of premium option* rider will cost $500, making for a total annual premium of $1,500. Assuming that you (the insured person) have no claims, or if your claims are less than 20% of total premiums paid during the period, you can expect to receive a refund of 70% of the premiums paid at the end of the tenth year of the policy, and every eighth year of the policy thereafter.

This type of rider normally pays out either on death or on expiry of the policy. In essence, it is a reward for staying healthy. In this hypothetical example, total premiums paid in the first 10 years would be $10,000 for the basic insurance plus $5,000 for the return of premium rider for a total cost of $15,000. At the end of 10 years, assuming there were no claims, the policyholder would receive a $10,500 refund of premiums.

This feature is useful for people who find it very hard to save and for those who like to feel that they are getting something for their insurance dollar. It does not make sense for those who already have an extremely tight cash flow. And of course, for those who make claims of over 20% of total premiums ($3,000 in the example given) the additional expense is not worthwhile.

Out of country claims

Some policies, especially so-called bare-bones policies, won't pay for claims outside Canada. People who travel a lot outside the country should examine potential policies carefully to ensure they have appropriate coverage for overseas claims.

War Exclusion

All policies have clauses stating that payments will not be made for claims arising from "war, insurrection," etc. In the wake of the September 11, 2001, terrorist attacks in New York, there was great concern that both life insurance claims and disability insurance claims arising as a result would not be honoured. In fact, all claims were honoured, but whether that will continue in the event of future attacks is debatable and will likely depend on the number of claims received.

Business Overhead Expense Rider; Key Person Disability Coverage

The *business overhead expense* or *key person disability* riders can be a part of a small business person's coverage so that if the owner or a key employee is disabled and cash flow is reduced, certain essential overhead expenses will be paid for under the policy. Key person disability coverage allows a small business to pay for a temporary worker to cover off the work normally performed in the company by the person with the disability. There are tax considerations in how these policies are structured. (See Chapter 10, "Disability and the Self-Employed Small Business Person.")

Tip: CompCorp provides Canadian life insurance policyholders with specified levels of protection against loss of benefits due to the financial failure (bankruptcy) of a Member Insurance Company. There are limits on coverage depending on the type of insurance. Disability Insurance is covered up to $2,000 per month of benefit. If you are considering purchasing more than this maximum coverage, consider splitting the coverage between two or more different insurance companies. It is important to ensure that both will pay out in the event of a claim, and that one company will not reduce (offset) payments based on payments from the other insurance company.

TAXATION ISSUES

The basic tax principles to remember with disability insurance are these:

- If the employee or individual pays for the premiums personally, then there is no tax on the benefits received if the person has a disability.
- If the employer pays for all or part of the premiums, as in company-sponsored benefits plans, then disability benefits when received by the employee will be totally or partly taxable.

Some employees take a short-sighted view of disability premium expenses when they see the premium cost being deducted from their pay. They assume that their employer is being cheap by not picking up the cost of the premium as an employee benefit. But at claims time, these same people would be angry if they were taxed on the benefits received!

One advantage to tax-free disability payments is that you need to purchase less disability insurance because no tax will be payable on payments from the policy.

But there are two disadvantages to tax-free disability benefits:

- The benefit payments, since they are not taxable, will not show up on your income tax return. This is not a problem unless you want to borrow money or move your mortgage to a different bank or financial institution. The first thing a financial institution will request is tax return assessments for the last 3 years to calculate your average annual income and assess your ability to handle the monthly payments. In the case of a long term disability, it is quite possible that the only income that will show up on your personal tax return is the Canada Pension Plan disability payments (if you qualify). These are not overly generous payments, and are not enough to qualify for much in the way of a loan and certainly not for the average mortgage. Financial institutions are not interested in non-taxable income, however substantial it may be. Proving that you have this income is not impossible, but it creates an additional headache.

- Disability insurance payments received, if they are taxable, are eligible as earned income for RRSP contribution limits. If, for example, a spouse is earning significant income, or there are other sources of income and there are significant savings each year, being able to tax shelter some of those savings in an RRSP on behalf of the person with the disability could be very useful in ensuring long term retirement income.

THE CLAIMS PROCESS

What Can The Policyholder Expect From The Insurance Company?

If you need to make a claim on your disability insurance, your first call will be to either the insurance company or to the agent who sold you the coverage. Insurance companies respond very quickly to claims as a rule. After submitting all the required documentation and assuming your claim is not *contestable*, you can expect to receive a letter stating the amount of benefit and when and how it will be paid. At this point, a *claims examiner* is assigned to your case. Normally, payments are direct-deposited to your bank account once a month after the waiting period has been satisfied.

The person with the disability or his or her representative *must be* familiar with the terms of the policy. If the original policy has been lost or mislaid, a new policy can be obtained from the insurance company upon payment of a small fee. If the claimant or the representative doesn't know what the terms and conditions are and what additional riders are on the policy, the insurance company may not honour them!

Contestable investigation

If a claim is made against the policy within 2 years of the date of policy purchase, there is almost always a *contestable investigation*, in case there was any misrepresentation on the policy application. Misrepresentation may be innocent (the applicant forgot to mention something that was materially important.) Or the misrepresentation may be fraudulent (misstating occupation, income, health and other factors.) In any event, an investigation is highly likely on a claim made within the first 2 years of insurance coverage.

A contestable investigation takes time. It involves the following steps undertaken by the insurance company:

- Obtaining a decoded summary of claims to provincial medicare for the previous 7 years

- Obtaining copies of all medical, hospital, doctors' and pharmacists' records
- Obtaining copies of 2 to 5 years of tax returns

Undisclosed information can work against you even if it does not relate to the cause of the current disability. In other words, failure to disclose that you were treated for stress in the past is significant, *even though* the disability claim relates to something else entirely.

Assessment of the claim

The next stage that the insurance company goes through is assessing the disability in relation to the policy.

- Has the disability continued beyond the elimination period before benefits are payable?
- Was the claim received within the filing period? This is normally 30 to 90 days after onset of disability, within a maximum of 1 year.
- What is the definition of total disability—regular occupation, own occupation, any occupation by virtue of training, education or experience?
- Is the disability a result of accident or sickness?
- What policy exclusions or waivers are there? For example, some policies do not cover mental disability or stress-related disability.
- Is the policy integrated with benefits from other sources, for example, CPP, workers' compensation?

Remember that *diagnosis does not equal disability.* You do not have a claim until the disability or disease reaches the point that you are unable to work any longer, as certified by a medical practitioner. The underwriters' understanding of the occupational requirements of a particular job is important in determining the claim.

About 10% to 20% of all new disability claims are related to mental and nervous conditions. It is estimated that up to 50% of total claims are in this category.

Ongoing assessments by medical personnel, whether by the disabled person's own physician or an in-house or independent medical professional hired by the insurance company, are required once the claim is in process and after it has been accepted.

Insurance companies not only do their own investigations when they believe there is a fraudulent claim, but they also rely on others to inform them—neighbours, insurance agents, and medical personnel who have come into contact with the claimant.

Janet's story

> *One month after filing the claim, the disability insurance carrier changed—the original company had sold its book of disability policies to another insurance company. However, the new carrier was prompt with payments, and the "waiver of premiums" rider kicked in, so that was one less monthly payment I had to make. The problems arose after I returned to work. I have "residual income benefits" and my income can fluctuate enormously month-to-month. I returned to work before I should have as it was tax season again and I knew I would have no business left if I didn't return that year. So after reducing the workload dramatically, and informing the insurance company, I started working again. At about the same time, the claims examiner changed, and the new one didn't seem to know how to handle residual income benefits. There was no communication, no information on what I needed to provide to them each month and an attitude that I must be malingering!*
>
> *I waited months for cheques at times despite numerous phone calls from me and my broker, and things only improved after I paid a lawyer to write a letter on my behalf. Since then, I have had three other claims examiners—four different ones in 10 months! For the third year, I am fighting to get the Cost of Living Adjustment applied.*

I have not been impressed with the accounting or accountability at all, but my concern is more that others without a financial background such as I have may not be receiving all the benefits to which they are entitled. I have found the Ombudsman's office at the insurance company to be very helpful, though, and they at least voiced concern about what was going on. The relationship that the public has with insurance companies is an interesting one—as long as there isn't a claim, they like to be perceived as our best friends. But the minute there is a claim, we have to recognize that the relationship shifts to an adversarial one and we are on opposite sides.

What is the Role of the Insurance Agent?

At the time of purchase, the agent or broker was paid a commission by the insurance company. As long as the policy remains in force, the insurance company pays the agent a small administrative fee each year. When a person has a claim, the first call should be to the agent who sold the insurance. The agent can then get involved in the following ways:

- Assisting with completing and filing the required initial claim forms, which can be very long and complex in some cases
- Gathering the requested information
- Explaining the contract in detail and the claims process to the client
- Informing claimants, if the claim is in the first 2 years of the policy being in force, of the contestable investigation
- Explaining the importance of filing all the requested information as soon as possible
- Participating in the appeals process and acting as an advocate with the insurance company.

The insurance agent's role is an interesting one. Although the insurance company is paying the agent, the *duty of care* the agent owes to the client is substantial. Some agents will be actively involved in the process; others choose to have minimal involvement. Insurance agents are not normally sent copies of all correspondence with the claimant, and authorization by the claimant must be given to the insurance company in writing to allow the agent to share in all confidential client information. Even then, the insurance company may answer only the agent's questions and not volunteer information.

Some claims departments actively discourage agent or broker involvement when there is a claim. They may feel that the agent will help the client to claim the most— and a good agent probably would. Another issue is that some lawyers are now advising agents to stay out of the claims process because of potential claims against the agents' errors and omissions insurance. When considering purchasing an individual policy, you should question the agent as to whether he/she will assist you if you have a claim.

What Happens if there are Problems in the Claims Process?

As with all businesses, service can vary from company to company and even among individuals within the company. The insurance company from which coverage was purchased may have sold its book of business to a different company; the insurance agent may have retired. This can be irritating for the person making a claim, but claims are normally honoured without difficulty.

If there are ongoing problems with the insurance company, there are sources of information and support.

The Canadian Life and Health Insurance Association (CLHIA) attempts to resolve problems consumers have with their life and disability policies, when claims have been denied. They also have an OmbudService to help resolve problems beyond the initial complaint stage handled through the Consumer Assistance Centre. In addition, they can provide the name and direct telephone number of the ombudsperson at each of the insurance companies. The role of this ombudsperson is to deal with problems that people claiming benefits may face, such as cheques not being received in a timely fashion or other issues.

Speaking from Experience...

Anita's story

I had paid into an employer-sponsored plan with the public service for about 8 years before starting my new job at the hospital. They very kindly waived the 3-month waiting period on the extended health benefits, but they were unable to do so for the disability coverage. Just under 3-months into the job, I was in the hospital with a spinal arteriovenous malformation. If I had still been at the Ministry, I would have had 75% of my salary for the first 6 months while I was on short-term disability and then, if I needed to be on long term disability, I would have had two thirds of my salary for as long as I was disabled, as well as partial disability benefits as I slowly returned to work.

As it was, I had EI of $300 per week for the first 15 weeks and then CPP disability. That was a bit of a shock actually, CPP told me that disability benefits weren't available on an "interim" basis— that you had to be totally and permanently disabled. At that point, I was not prepared to admit that there was any permanent disability. But the staff at the rehabilitation hospital persuaded me that I was going to have permanent effects in my life and that I met the criteria for CPP disability. I did therefore receive CPP disability at the maximum of about $960 per month, plus some payments for the children each month.

I must say that I did not have a bad experience with CPP, and that I found them to be very supportive. I learned that, under the new policies, you can go back to work for 3 months and if it doesn't work out, you can go back on to CPP. This is what happened to me—I tried to go back to work too soon, in my state of denial. That's the good news—the bad news is that you couldn't live on a CPP disability pension in Toronto. The situation was compounded by the fact that my husband, to whom I'd only been married a few months when this all happened, had just become self-employed prior to all this happening. Poor guy—I was supposed to be the one with a stable income while he started his own business.

What's the alternative? If we are going to have insurance companies which, when you change jobs, are allowed to deny you coverage for the first 3 months, there is a huge gap here that is not being covered. And yet to take out individual coverage, and pay monthly premiums so that in effect you are protected twice for the same risk except when you are between jobs, seems like a huge financial burden and one that most people simply cannot afford.

What we need is a public system that provides more extensive coverage than CPP. The alternative may be for insurance companies to provide coverage that starts immediately at the beginning of a new job, even if the employee must pay higher premiums the first 3 months; or that a prior employer's disability insurance plan will cover an employee for 3 months after they have left their job. It should be portable, like pensions are now.

I felt and I still feel, that I had paid thousands of dollars for long term disability insurance over the years and when I needed it I could not access it. It seems to me that there is something basically wrong with a system that functions in this way.

Comments from an Insurance agent

When you get a job and the employer asks the insurance company to waive the waiting period (usually 3 months) normally *all* benefits start at the same time. I have never heard of everything except the Long term disability starting immediately. This must be a special provision of their policy. Employers will sometimes ask me if the waiting period can be eliminated for a specific employee that they have hired, and I tell them yes, with a letter to the insurance company. I think the hospital [as employer] slipped up here. It is the employer who drives the group insurance and it is up to the employer to request the benefits they require and when those benefits are to commence from the insurance company. The LTD waiting period was a provision of the policy and the employer could have waived it. If not, they should have been looking for a new insurance company. Insurance companies do not make the rules of a 3-month wait, the employer *chooses*. Most employers do use 3 months just so they don't have to pay for employees who don't stay with them. However, it is still the employer's choice. They can have a zero waiting period if they want, or they could choose 1 month. The onus is on the employer not the insurance company.

John's story

When I got the settlement, I was receiving a disability pension from my union. When I got the settlement, the union cut off my disability pension. Apparently in their contract, it stated that if you get a settlement or income from any other source, you are not entitled to the disability pension any more. This went on for many years, and then I realized that my other money was not going to last me forever, so I managed to find another lawyer who was prepared to take my case. I got a back settlement of $65,000 of which $20,000 went to the lawyer, and all of it is taxable. But I wasn't so much concerned about the back payments as I was about receiving a monthly *income for the rest of my life. The pension is $1300 per month. I felt very angry about the whole thing—after all, I had paid into this for years, and I felt that the pension is something I am entitled to and I still feel that way. It really is a game they play—when it comes down to it, nobody wants to pay the money.*

SOURCES OF INFORMATION

The Canadian Life and Health Insurance Association (CLHIA) has a Consumer Assistance Centre at 1-800-268-8099; in Toronto the number is 416-777-2344; web site at www.clhia.ca.

The Web site for CompCorp is www.compcorp.ca. This is the agency that provides protection for insurance benefits.

To contact a lawyer specializing in disability insurance issues, a referral from someone who has had a similar problem and who was pleased with the results is always best, or contact your Provincial Law Society.

GLOSSARY

CPP offset: Provision in some group disability policies that states that disability benefits received by an insured person under a group policy are reduced by the dollar amount of CPP disability benefits the insured person also receives. See also "Integration".

Elimination period: Number of days (sometimes number of days plus other conditions) that must elapse before a certain type of insurance policy will begin paying out benefits to the insured. Also called the "Waiting Period".

Integration: Provision in some individual or group disability policies that states that the benefit payout under the policy will be reduced by (integrated with) the dollar amount of benefits received from other disability insurance payors, such as other group disability plans or workers' compensation plans. See also "CPP Offset".

Morbidity: The possibility that in a population, certain individuals will develop illnesses or diseases or will suffer non-fatal accidents.

Partial disability: The condition of disability from injury or illness that leaves the insured person not totally disabled, but which means that the insured is unable to work at least 50% of the time and is unable to perform one or more of the important duties or his or her occupation.

Policyholder: Person for whom insurance coverage is provided. Also known as plan holder or insured, provided that the individual is also the recipient of any insurance benefits payable.

Premium: The fee that is paid to insurance companies to maintain a particular type of insurance policy on behalf of an individual (or a group if the employer is paying the cost).

Residual income benefits: Provision in disability insurance policy. Provides benefit payments to insured based on benchmarks of income earned by the insured as they begin to return to work on a gradual basis. Allows insured to earn certain levels of income while continuing to receive specified amounts of disability benefit payments.

Rider: An optional, contractual provision added to an insurance policy that amends the policy by adding or decreasing benefits or waiving certain coverage. Example: Waiver of Premium on Disability rider.

Total disability: The condition of disability from injury or illness that is extreme and that results in the loss of earned income over a certain percentage (usually over 75%) and requires a certain level of medical or other care.

Underwriting: Criteria used by insurance companies to determine those groups or individuals they will cover for particular types of insurance based on risk factors. Also, process of spreading risk, by which insurance is provided on behalf of corporate/group sponsors for their members or employees.

Waiting period: See "Elimination Period".

CHAPTER 5

EMPLOYEE BENEFIT AND INDIVIDUAL PLANS: EXTENDED HEALTH AND OPTIONAL INSURANCE

Employee benefit plan is the term that refers to all the benefits offered to employees either on a cost-shared basis or an employer-paid basis. Extended health care benefits, short-term and long term disability benefits, life insurance, accidental death and dismemberment insurance and critical illness insurance can all form part of these group packages. Long term care insurance is an add-on benefit, especially in some group retirement plans.

The "cafeteria style benefits" described in some employee benefit booklets mean that employees can mix and match benefits to suit themselves and their families. Be careful. For example, don't drop disability coverage in favour of a vision care option that allows you and your family to have glasses every 2 years. The risk of disability is potentially more serious than the cost of eyeglasses!

EXTENDED HEALTH BENEFITS

Extended health benefits coverage, also known as *supplementary health insurance*, is important to Canadians. Why? Because provincial health care systems provide only basic medical care for Canadians and not all health expenses are covered. If you want extra coverage, or coverage on optional items, you have to obtain it on your own. Most provinces do not cover the following items, or cover for a limited period or only up to a certain value:

- Dental care
- Medications and prescriptions (sometimes seniors or welfare recipients are covered)

- Glasses and contact lenses
- Ambulance services
- Medical equipment and supplies, prosthetics
- Specialized treatments or services (e.g., extensive physiotherapy, home nursing)

Think of extended health benefits as a means to enhance or top up provincial health plans. The main concerns for most people are drug and medication expenses, vision care and dental care coverage. Consequently, most plans offer these coverage options.

Where Do You Get Extended Health Benefits and Optional Insurance Coverage?

- Through your employer's plan
- Through your own private plan
- Through an affinity group (e.g., Chamber of Commerce, alumni group, professional association, through a bank on a loan or credit card.)

Group or employer extended health benefit plans

Most Canadians have extended health benefits and supplementary health benefits through their employers. Many employers are now restricting such coverage because the level of claims has soared in recent years.

In the Globe and Mail, Paulette Peirol reported that some employers estimate that their plan costs for drugs rise by about 8% per year. Drug costs account for between 70 to 90% of a private health care plan costs. Part of the reason for the increase in drug costs, according to a study by Green Shield Canada, is a combination of the following factors:

- Demographics—an aging population requiring medication
- Physicians prescribing new drugs that are more expensive (but don't necessarily work better than the old ones), because the pharmaceutical companies have marketed them extensively. New

drugs account for more than 45% of the total cost of drug claims.

- Drugs used as preventive agents
- Patent laws that prevent the prescription of cheaper generic drugs

The fall of corporate profits in the past few years means that employers are looking for ways to reduce their costs. And reducing benefit costs is a major area of scrutiny by human resource departments and senior management. In many cases, they achieve cuts by limiting drug coverage to generic drugs or those that have been on the market for many years, as opposed to newer, more expensive drugs that the pharmaceutical companies are marketing to doctors. Often, if a new drug is prescribed, the doctor must explain why the new drug is required, instead of an already established drug, before the patient can be reimbursed. Sometimes, the plans will not cover costs of new drugs. In many cases, it is worthwhile to talk with a pharmacist about the relative differences between a new drug and an older, established drug—especially if the extended health benefit plan will not cover the new drug. New does not necessarily mean better: the older drugs have a performance history with patients; new drugs do not. There may be side effects from the new drugs that are yet unknown.

Whether your employer provides extended health benefits or whether you buy them privately, there are a number of choices. Think of extended health benefits as a "buffet" of benefits. Some employers allow employees to pick and choose their benefits and optional insurance, of which extended health benefits may be a part, up to a certain number of points or a dollar value. There are cheap employer plans that offer little or no choice, and there are top-of-the-line plans that offer many mix and match opportunities.

If your family has two wage earners with extended health coverage, read the plans carefully and select options from each that offer the most value. For example, one plan may reimburse dental expenses at an 80% rate of the provincial dental fee chart from 3 years previous, whereas the other plan may reimburse at a rate of 80% of current year rates. By combining the coverage under both plans, families can get 100% coverage on dental claims (and in other areas as well). Read the fine print carefully and check with the human resources or benefits office to make sure that you submit claims correctly.

> **Tip:** Extended health benefit premiums paid by the employee are considered as medical expenses and qualify for the medical expense tax credit on your income tax return. Self-employed individuals and incorporated businesses can deduct extended health benefit premiums as a business expense. (See Chapter 10, "Disability And The Self-Employed Small Business Person.")

Privately purchased extended health benefits plans

Private plans also offer a "buffet" of choices and price points. The plans essentially offer the same types of coverage as group plans. The difference is that with private plans, individuals must pay for their own coverage.

As with other kinds of insurance, companies are concerned about pre-existing conditions. Fortunately, to join most large employer-sponsored plans, you will not need a medical and you likely will not be excluded because you have a pre-existing condition. The insurance companies' concerns about pre-existing conditions are taken care of in the pricing models that they use for these large plans. In these large plans, a new employee with a disability can expect to receive all the same benefits as other employees, including coverage for prescription drugs related to his or her disability, if they are on the list of covered medications under that plan. Smaller employer plans, however, such as those with fewer than 10 employees, will often require the completion of a questionnaire, and pre-existing conditions disclosed may be excluded from the employee's coverage.

Pre-existing medical conditions are very important if you are buying extended health benefits on your own. If you have had heart problems, cancer, degenerative discs, or indeed, have ever seen a specialist for something as simple as acne treatment, then the insurance company insists that these conditions must be disclosed on your application. You will either be denied coverage on these medical problem areas, or your premiums will be raised to reflect the higher risk the insurance company undertakes to cover certain of these areas. Failure to disclose pre-existing conditions on an extended health benefits application means that, if you make a claim for payment related to that condition in the future, the insurance company could reject it.

Janet's story

I had purchased my private extended health benefit plan 15 years before my accident. The medical questionnaire asked for the names of all doctors I had consulted within the previous 5 years. As I saw a chiropractor regularly as a preventative measure, my policy stated that anything to do with my spine was not covered! I never dreamt that I would have an accident and break my neck and so never thought too much about it. My insurance agent went to bat for me with the insurance company and they did cover my semi-private hospital and so on, but it took several weeks and lots of medical reports before it was cleared up. My advice—if an exclusion is put on that is too restrictive, then appeal it or look elsewhere for coverage.

Travel Insurance

Travel insurance is a form of supplementary health insurance that is primarily for people travelling abroad.

All provinces have a cap on provincial health care coverage if you are away from Canada for more than a certain number of days. For example, in Ontario, there is no provincial coverage (OHIP) if the person has been out of Canada for more than 214 days. The exception is if he or she is a student attending an overseas university as part of full-time education and has had prior approval from the provincial medicare administrators. Someone who has been absent from Canada for more than 214 days (not just students) may be treated as a new resident upon their return and may not be able to obtain coverage under provincial plans for 3 months. If you are going to be away from Canada for more than 214 days, you need a different type of travel insurance for coverage after the 214 days have expired.

Canadians moving from one province to another have coverage from their province of origin for 3 months after leaving that province, at which time the new province of residence provides coverage. This does not apply to students moving to another province to attend university. New residents moving to Canada from another country are not usually eligible for coverage until they have been resident in a Canadian province for 3 months.

Travel insurance is often used to fill the gap before a new Canadian becomes eligible for provincial health care coverage. Most travel insurance is available only up to the end of the medicare waiting-period, which is 3 months. At the end of the 3-month period, if a person still cannot obtain provincial coverage, a different type of policy will be required. Consult with an insurance specialist.

Travel insurance coverage may be part of an employer plan or it can be purchased privately.

Coverage typically includes the following features:

- Payment for the cost of air ambulance or other transportation to a treatment facility out of the country
- Payment up to a certain dollar value for emergency medical treatment
- Payment for hotel and other expenses for accompanying person
- Payment for repatriation (return) to Canada for the patient and accompanying person

When buying individual policies, the important things to look out for are as follows:
- As high a dollar limit on the policy as possible and preferably unlimited.
- A minimal number of exclusions. (Read the exclusions carefully.)
- A clear explanation of the policy terms on pre-existing conditions. A claim may be denied for non-disclosure even if the pre-existing condition is not the cause of a claim.

There is also coverage available for Visitors to Canada and for International Students in Canada.

Read the fine print carefully!

OTHER INSURANCE COVERAGE

Many group plans, especially employee benefit plans, incorporate not only extended health insurance, but also life and disability insurance and, in some cases, critical illness and long term care insurance. Some larger companies offer employees a selection of benefits ranging from orthodontics to a higher level of disability insurance or additional life insurance. Employees are given a dollar amount or a number of points to be allocated as they wish to the different benefit options. Typically the number of points available rises with length of service and sometimes with salary level.

Be sure to insure the basics before using points to purchase more costly benefits such as extended health. Forgoing disability coverage in favour of family vision care may mean that you see dollars coming in regularly, but in the event of a disability, you may have little or no coverage.

Although the coverage you choose will depend on your situation and family needs, you should consider the following benefits as essential, in order of importance:

- Maximum disability benefits
- Life insurance coverage; consider increasing the amount especially if you have dependents
- Spousal coverage, if applicable
- Extended health benefits

Other Group Benefits Available

Group and individual plans offer other benefits as well. A *family transportation benefit* can be particularly useful for Canadians who do not live near a large urban centre or need to go to another province for treatment. If you need major rehabilitation in a hospital setting or residential facility, or if you need specialized treatment, a typical plan may pay *reasonable* hotel expenses for your family and transportation *by the most direct route* to visit you in the hospital. Generally, the limit on this kind of coverage is less than $5,000 and requires that the patient's residence be at least 150 kilometres from the hospital or treatment facility.

Another benefit that may be available is the *home alteration and vehicle modification* benefit. This pays for modifications to your home to make it wheelchair accessible and modifications to a vehicle. All these types of expenses must be required modifications and must be as a result of sustaining a *covered loss*. A *covered loss* is normally one that results in a medical professional certifying that the modifications are required as a result of the patient's condition.

Extended health benefits may also provide coverage for mobility devices in the event of a mobility impairment, for example, wheelchairs and walkers.

(For more on equipment, see Chapter 15, "Attendant Care Services and Equipment Funding.")

There are many other types of benefits that may be available in different plans. Familiarize yourself with the benefits in your own plan and get as much information as possible before purchasing an individual plan.

The following table illustrates the variety of options that may be available. Not all of these options will be available in all plans.

OPTIONS FOR EMPLOYEE AND GROUP BENEFIT PLANS

FEATURE OR BENEFIT	TYPICAL CONDITIONS AND LIMITATIONS
In-hospital Upgrade Benefit	May be able to purchase upgrade to semi-private or private room, usually for a maximum number of days per year up to a maximum dollar value, e.g., $150 or $200 per day.
Hospital Benefits (cash payments)	May be combined with hospital upgrade coverage. Cash amount paid to patient every day they are in hospital to cover miscellaneous expenses. May be $50, $100 per day. Usually a lifetime maximum e.g., 1,000 days.
Short Term Disability or Sickness Plan	Depending on the plan, benefits range from 15, 17, 26, to 52 weeks. May be reduced by Employment Insurance Sick Benefits.
Long Term Disability Plan	May cover rehabilitation costs, workplace modification. May be for partial or full disability. May require return to work after a certain number of years. May be taxable or non-taxable. (See Chapter 4, Disability Insurance.)
Long Term Disability Plan Specialized Coverages	Specialty coverage offered by some insurance companies: (a) Overage Worker, e.g., people over age 60 or over age 65 who are still working; (b) High Net Worth or

FEATURE OR BENEFIT	TYPICAL CONDITIONS AND LIMITATIONS
	those with high levels of unearned income from investments; (c) Non-Standard Occupations, e.g., entertainers; (d) Offshore Employees, e.g., those working in the Middle East or Asia; (e) Partner Buy-out, if a partner in an enterprise becomes disabled, others can buy him or her out; (f) Disability coverage for employees who have been downsized and have therefore lost their disability coverage from their former employer
Dental Care	Usually covers basic preventive care and maintenance: check-ups, cleanings, X-rays, fillings, extractions, some root canal procedures. Enhanced plans cover root canals, crowns, bridges, orthodontics. How often you can see your dentist in a year varies from 6 to 9 months. Reimbursement is up to certain percentage of provincial dental fee table, e.g., 70% or 80%. Some plans limit maximum costs per year per family or individual. May be deductible fee charged. Predetermination forms required for certain procedures or insurance company might not pay.
Accidental Dental Care	Maximum dollar amount per year, e.g., $1,000 or $2,000.
Prescription Drugs and Medications	Some plans pay only for generic drugs prescribed; top-up plans allow for brand name drug prescriptions. A limited dollar amount may be payable per year. Payment is percentage of cost of drugs up to maximum per year, e.g., 70%, 100%. May be cap on dispensing fees. May be age limits by certain insurance companies.
Accidental Death and Dismemberment	Covers loss of, or loss of use of limbs, sight, etc. Amount payable depends upon the principal amount covered under the plan: payment is a percentage of that principal depending upon the loss. (Loss of life =100% payout, as does loss of or loss of use of both hands or both feet or sight in both eyes.)

FEATURE OR BENEFIT	TYPICAL CONDITIONS AND LIMITATIONS
Vision Care	Dollar value maximum. May be every 2 or 3 years that glasses or contact lenses can be covered.
Travel Coverage	Trips up to certain maximum number of days, e.g., 15, 30 days per trip; coverage for emergency hospital and medical care; pre-existing conditions may be excluded from coverage. Enhanced plans may offer $1 million per person per trip. May offer baggage or air flight or common carrier coverage, trip cancellation insurance, etc., repatriation of deceased, diagnostic services such as laboratory tests.
Hearing Aids	Dollar maximum for purchase and repair of hearing aid over stated time frame, e.g., $500 per 36 consecutive months.
Ambulance services	Dollar maximum for ambulance costs over provincial payout. Covers ground or air ambulance, e.g., $1,000 per year.
Medical Equipment, Assistive Devices and Prosthetics	Dollar maximum per year, e.g., wheelchair rental up to $2,500 per year; dollar maximum per year for artificial limbs and other assistive devices, e.g., up to $2,500 per year.
Home Nursing Care	Maximum dollar value per year for Registered Nurse, or Health Care Aide, or equivalent, e.g., up to $2,500 or $5,000 per year.
Specialized Medical or Health Care Professionals: Physiotherapist Occupational Therapist Osteopath Psychologist Speech Therapist Chiropodist/Podiatrist Chiropractor Massage Therapist Homeopath/Naturopath Private Care Nurse	Each insurance company has certain set maximums for the number of appointments covered and the dollar value of costs covered. Sometimes the reimbursement is based on a certain amount for an initial visit, with another dollar amount for subsequent visits. Usually, the benefits start only after the provincial yearly maximums for such services are reached. (In some provinces, not all these specialists are covered by the provincial health care plan.) There may also be waiting periods before benefits start.

FEATURE OR BENEFIT	TYPICAL CONDITIONS AND LIMITATIONS
Long Term Care Benefits	Available as benefit on some employer plans or as private coverage. Pays out benefits subject to per day dollar maximum based on policy if policyholder requires at home care or nursing home care.
Critical Illness Coverage	Lump sum payment made if policyholder suffers certain medical conditions as outlined in contract. Usually there is a waiting period before benefit will be paid out (as a lump sum). Benefit amount may be reduced as person moves into older age bracket. Pre-existing conditions excluded from coverage. Coverage may end at certain age – e.g., 64, 65 or 70. Spouse and dependents can be covered.
Critical Illness Coverage – Treatment in United States and Abroad	Lump-sum maximums higher than regular Critical Illness policies; maximum amount from $350,000 to $1 million for medical care outside of Canada. If policyholder has one of a list of covered ailments, then Best Doctors™ gives clinical guidance in diagnosis and treatment plan and directs patient to best care option. Available through some employer plans, also through private plan.
Family Transportation Benefit	For patients whose families do not live near the hospital or rehab centre. Provides hotel accommodation and transportation benefit to patient's family if normal residence is certain number of kilometres from hospital; dollar maximum, e.g., 150 kilometres, no more than $5,000.
Home Alteration & Vehicle Modification Benefit	Pays dollar amount to modify home to make it wheelchair accessible and to modify vehicle for same purpose. Must be required modifications and specifically covered in policy. (Separate from amounts payable through provincial or charitable programs.)

Not all policies will have all the options listed above, nor will all allow for combining of certain coverages. Some insurance companies will have *preset option packages*. Still others will only allow certain options to be purchased as *stand-alone coverage*. Each insurance company will offer different options, different coverage levels, and different premiums. Shop around very carefully and very extensively to get what you need.

Tip: CompCorp provides Canadian life insurance policyholders with specified levels of protection against loss of benefits due to the financial failure of a Member Insurance Company. There are limits on coverage depending on the type of insurance. Travel Insurance Benefits and Extended Health Insurance Benefits are each guaranteed to a lump-sum maximum of $60,000.

ACCIDENTAL DEATH AND DISMEMBERMENT INSURANCE

People who need life insurance should first buy adequate ordinary life insurance, which pays out at death from most causes. As the name implies, Accidental Death coverage only pays out if death occurs as the result of an accident. Statistically, this is not as likely as death from other causes.

Accidental death and dismemberment insurance is a potential source of funds for those who have become disabled through an accident or sudden disabling illness. Of concern to a person with the disability, of course, is the *dismemberment* provision of the policy. *Dismemberment* is usually defined as loss of use of a limb or limbs, or the actual severing of a limb or limbs. Therefore, a person with paraplegia who has lost the use of both legs would qualify for payment under this definition. Depending upon the policy, the sum involved may be substantial.

Although accidental death and dismemberment insurance is not a top priority for insurance purchasers, it is often included in private life insurance policies or in group benefit plans as an adjunct to life insurance coverage, as well as in affinity plans such as alumni, business and professional association, bank and credit card plans. It should not be overlooked as a potential source of funds by people with disabilities or their representatives.

Some employee benefit plans also include definitions of *critical diseases* that cause the loss of or loss of use of limbs, and therefore, provide insurance payouts. For example, one employee group benefit plan includes this coverage:

> If the employee sustains one of the following losses, as a direct result of Critical Disease or resulting directly and independently of other causes from bodily injuries occasioned solely through external, violent and accidental means, without negligence on the employee's part, the insurance company will pay:
> An amount equal to 200% of the basic life insurance for
> - Paraplegia (total paralysis of both lower limbs), or
> - Hemiplegia (total paralysis of one side of the body), or
> - Quadriplegia (total paralysis of all four limbs).
>
> An amount equal to 100% of the amount of basic life insurance for
> - Loss of both hands or of both feet, or
> - Loss of the sight of both eyes, or
> - Loss of one hand and one foot, or
> - Loss of use of both hands, or
> - Loss of use of both arms, or
> - Loss of use of both legs, or
> - Loss of use of one hand or arm and one leg, or
> - Loss of sight of one eye and one hand or one foot.

This particular plan also provides additional coverage. It will pay 50% of the amount of the basic life insurance coverage if there is the loss of, or loss of use of, one limb or eye or hand. It will pay 33.3% of the amount of basic life insurance if there is a lesser amount of loss, such as the loss of certain fingers of the hand, loss of speech, or hearing.

Each insurance company has different definitions; each company will have different provisions before they will pay out on a claim. For example, the policy states that "loss of hand shall mean severance at or above the wrist"; "paralysis shall mean complete and irreversible paralysis caused by brain, spine, muscle or nerve damage as a result of an accident or Covered Critical Disease, which has continued for a period of 12 months from the date of the accident or diagnosis or critical illness."

Consult a knowledgeable insurance specialist before buying any kind of insurance.

CHECKLIST FOR EXTENDED HEALTH BENEFITS/ SUPPLEMENTARY HEALTH BENEFITS AND OPTIONAL INSURANCE COVERAGE

- ✔ What coverage do you need? For example, a young family may want dental coverage, whereas an older couple may be more interested in having drug plan coverage and critical illness or long term care insurance.
- ✔ Have you prioritized the coverage needed? For example, be sure to retain disability coverage as you select coverage from a "buffet" of benefits offered by an employer plan.
- ✔ What are the maximum dollar values covered under a certain plan? For example, most plans limit the dollar value of reimbursement for eyeglasses or contact lenses to a stated amount every 2 or 3 years.
- ✔ What is the premium cost of the coverage?
- ✔ What are the deductibles for coverage? Some plans require that a certain deductible amount be paid each year per family; for example, you pay the first

$75 before the drug plan coverage starts for the year.

- ✔ What amount of co-insurance is required? In short, what percentage of eligible expenses over your deductible is payable by you? Typically, it is 10% or 20%, but it may be as high as 50% for certain major dental procedures.
- ✔ What can you afford?
- ✔ Do you know how to claim from the benefit plans of both working spouses so that maximum coverage can be obtained? (Remember, the amount of reimbursement cannot exceed 100% of the cost of the expenses incurred.)
- ✔ Is there a medical questionnaire required?
- ✔ Are there pre-existing conditions that are excluded from coverage?
- ✔ Is there an age limit to the benefits you want?
- ✔ Can the employer benefits be topped up by private plan coverage of choice?
- ✔ To what extent can you self-insure, that is, do you have enough assets and/or income to cover all your needs, including potential dental and medical costs? And to what extent does paying premiums for coverage make economic sense?
- ✔ How secure are the benefits from change by the insurance company? Is it likely that your coverage will be reduced or changed by the employer in the near future? Would private benefits in a certain area be more secure?
- ✔ If losing your job or leaving your job is a possibility, have you checked out possible coverage through a private plan? To what extent can you convert your group extended health benefits into a private plan for which you pay yourself if you leave your employer?
- ✔ If you are near retirement, which employer plan benefits will continue in your retirement? For

those benefits that will not continue, shop around to find private replacement coverage before your retirement date!

✔ For private extended health benefit coverage, how many insurance companies have you checked out? Shopping around, with the help of a knowledgeable insurance agent, is critical.

✔ If you have a claim, remember that most plans require that the claim be started within 1 year after the eligible expenses are incurred or the event that triggered a claim (e.g., an accident) occurred.

✔ Extended health plan premiums are a medical expense for tax purposes. For self-employed and incorporated businesses they are a business expense.

SOURCES OF INFORMATION:

Canadian Life and Health Insurance Association (CLHIA): www.clhia.ca Go to Consumer Assistance Centre button on the site. Information on extended health benefit insurance companies.

Canadian Institute for Health Information (CIHI): www.cihi.ca for information on health care expenditures in Canada.

Specific insurance companies and distributors have Web sites or can be contacted through a qualified life and health insurance agent. (See also CLHIA above.)

The Globe and Mail, Toronto, Friday, April 18, 2003, article, *"Benefits in sick bay"*, by Paulette Peirol.

See Chapter 10, "Disability and the Self-employed Small Businessperson" for information on Personal Health Services Plans.

CHAPTER 6

CRITICAL ILLNESS INSURANCE AND LONG TERM CARE INSURANCE

Obtaining disability insurance should be the priority for working people; if it is not possible to obtain disability insurance, then critical illness insurance should be considered. If you are looking for disability, critical illness, or long term care insurance coverage and have ever been disabled or diagnosed with any one of a long list of conditions, you may find coverage very hard to obtain. There are many factors taken into account, such as the type of condition and length of time since there has been any recurrence of the problem. There are insurance brokers who specialize in obtaining coverage for people who are hard to insure, but the costs of coverage may be very high.

Always consult an insurance professional with expertise in *disability, critical illness, and long term care insurance* before making any insurance decisions related to income replacement or income supplement plans.

CRITICAL ILLNESS INSURANCE

Disability insurance is the basic building block of coverage for most working Canadians. It provides an income, for the period of time covered by the contract, which replaces a portion of the income that has been cut off because of disability.

But what about people who do not work? What about those who are out of the workforce because they are caring for a child or another family member with a disability? What about those who are homemakers or who are retired? Or those who are not yet eligible for disability insurance, such as new business owners?

What about large, lump-sum expenses, which even those covered by disability income payments, cannot cover from cash flow? A solution that may work for these individuals is *critical illness insurance.*

Critical illness insurance is a relatively new kid on the insurance block: it has been available in Canada only since 1992. Available in Europe for many years, it accounts for 20% of all personal insurance policies sold in Europe, as compared with fewer than 4% of all Canadian personal insurance policies sold.

What is Critical Illness Insurance?

As opposed to an income based on pre-disability working income, critical illness benefits are paid out as a one-time, lump-sum payment. The payout is made only if you develop a *life-threatening* form of one of up to two dozen medical ailments.

Of course, the willingness of an insurance company to insure you depends upon the company's research into your health. Your family health history may mean that you are not a desirable risk for the insurance company. There may be extra premium costs, or you may simply be declined coverage.

Critical illness plans offered by some companies may be combined with other types of coverage, such as disability policies or life insurance policies.

How Does Critical Illness Insurance Work?

The funds paid out from a critical illness insurance policy can be used as the policyholder sees fit. The exception is *medical treatment critical illness policies* that enable policyholders to obtain more expensive treatment (often in the United States) up to a certain dollar value instead of a lump-sum payout on diagnosis. Although the premiums in the latter type of policy may be lower than a regular critical illness policy, the flexibility and, indeed, the necessity for payout may be lower, too.

Benefits received from a regular critical illness policy have no restrictions on how they can be spent. They can be used to:

- Pay off the mortgage or other personal debt
- Pay for medical treatments not covered by government or private health insurance
- Pay for renovations to the home required as a result of the illness
- Pay for motor vehicle modifications
- Replace income lost as a result of time off work
- Ensure the survival of a small business
- Pay for a vacation, pay for children's education, or any other goals

What Does Critical Illness Insurance Cover?

Critical illness insurance covers life-threatening illnesses named in the policy. The key point is that if the *diagnosis* of a medical ailment indicates that it is *life threatening, and* it is on the list of ailments covered under the policy, then the policy must pay out the lump sum agreed upon in the contract.

Insurance companies have a list of basic ailments that are covered. These usually include:

- Cancer
- Heart Attack
- Stroke

Additional conditions, normally found in *enhanced critical illness* policies, vary according to the insurance companies' policies. These conditions may include the following:

- Organ transplants; organ failure
- Heart bypass surgery
- Kidney failure
- Paralysis
- Multiple sclerosis

- Blindness
- Deafness
- Alzheimer's disease
- Parkinson's disease
- Coma
- Speech loss
- Loss of limbs
- Major burns
- Brain tumours (benign)

These conditions are normally found in *Enhanced Critical Illness Policies*.

Definitions of covered illnesses

It is very important to understand the *definition* of the particular medical condition covered under the policy. Each insurance company will have its own definition of the condition that leads to a successful claim. The chart below illustrates the definition of *heart attack* by three different insurance companies.

The point to remember is this: know what the definitions of each medical condition are in the policy you take out. As insurance companies' experience with critical illness insurance matures, many specialists predict that there will be standardized definitions for critical illness insurance policies that will be updated by distributors every few years, as is the case in the United Kingdom.

Illness	Company 1	Company 2	Company 3
Heart Attack	Yes, covered	Yes, as shown by ECG changes and elevation of cardiac enzymes	Yes, as shown by ECG changes, elevation of cardiac enzymes, and chest pain

Policy Options, Riders, and Exclusions

In addition to paying out a lump sum, critical illness policies can be enhanced with policy riders or additions to coverage.

Return of premium

The return of premium option, for which insurance companies charge an additional premium, means that, if the policyholder person dies during the time the policy is in force and has never had a critical illness claim under the policy, some or all of the premiums paid will be returned to the policyholder's estate. This normally applies to *term to 75* and *term to 100 policies.* (The numbers in *term to 75* and *term to 100* refer to the age at which the policy ends.) If you decided to end coverage, known as *surrendering* the policy, before the end of the policy period, and you had no claims, then you would receive a return of premiums. But you would have paid extra for this feature.

Waiver of premium

The waiver of premium option means that if the policyholder becomes disabled (or the owner of the policy dies or becomes disabled, if the owner is someone other than the policyholder) there would be no premiums payable, but the policy coverage would continue.

Child rider

The child rider provides, that if the person who is insured dies, the policy will continue to cover the policyholder's children until they reach age 21, with no further premiums required. (This is referred to as a *paid-up benefit.*)

Exclusions

In addition to riders, insurance companies make other special rules that apply to their policies and that may result in claims being denied.

Insurance companies will not honour claims for disability or death under the following circumstances:

- When death or disability resulted from self-inflicted injury or suicide
- Claims as a result of war and hazards arising from war
- Disability or death resulting from the use of illegal or illicit drugs or the use of a drug, poisonous substance, intoxicant or narcotic unless prescribed by physician and taken in accordance with directions.
- Disability or death resulting from violation of criminal law
- Disability or death resulting from the operation of a motor vehicle while intoxicated beyond a certain point
- Injuries sustained while under the influence of alcohol
- When there is a diagnosis of cancer within 90 days of issue or reinstatement of a policy
- When the policyholder does not survive 30-day survival period from the date of diagnosis of the ailment
- Where there was a pre-existing condition
- When the policyholder has not been a resident of Canada for at least 1 year

Who is Eligible to Buy Critical Illness Insurance?

There's no *earned income* requirement for taking out critical illness insurance. This means that the insurance company looks at the following major factors before it will issue a policy to anyone.

What are the chances that the applicant will contract a covered critical illness?

The critical illness policy has a *survival period*. If the person who has a life-threatening ailment covered under the policy survives for a period of time (usually 30 days), then the policy pays out. The either/or nature of the policy condition for payout means that there is a higher rate of rejection for claims under critical illness policies than for other insurance claims. The rejection rate for critical illness insurance policy claims is 6%, as opposed to 4% for other policies, according to "The Insurance Journal," September 2001.

The survival period is one of the differences between disability insurance and critical illness insurance. Disability insurance is paid out if the individual cannot work after a certain waiting period. This means that a disability policy may not be paid out if the individual had a waiting period of, say, 6 months, and either recovered or died at the end of the 6-month period.

The insurance company therefore must look very carefully at your current and past health history and at your family health history. For example, if your family has a history of breast cancer or prostate cancer, then you may not be able to obtain coverage for that condition as part of the critical illness policy—or you may not be able to obtain critical illness coverage at all. Most companies require disclosure of a family history of such diseases as Alzheimer's disease, cancer, diabetes, high blood pressure, Huntington's chorea, kidney disease, mental illness or suicide, multiple sclerosis, stroke or any other inherited disease. You will be considered to be of higher risk if more than one family member has a history of a specific disease. Also important is the age of onset of the disease: the risk is higher the younger the family member was when he or she contracted the disease.

What is the age and sex of the person to be insured?

As with most insurance policies, the age of the applicant plays a role in the cost of the policy. The older the client, the higher the premium, because the possibility of a claim is higher.

The sex of the client determines a part of the potential risk, too. Based on their claims experience, the insurance company will set rates based on the claims history of men and women.

What Types of Critical Illness Plans are there?

There are several companies offering critical illness policies in Canada. The most common plans are:

- *Ten-year term insurance.* At the end of the term, a renewal of the policy is possible, usually up to an end period of age 75. Of course, at renewal, the policy price increases.
- *Level premium to age 75.* Depending upon the age at which the policy starts, the policy extends until age 75 with a fixed premium for the entire period.
- *Level premium to age 100.* The same conditions as age to 75, except that the policy expires at age 100.

How Much Does Critical Illness Insurance Cost?

Most critical illness policies are non-cancellable, which means that the policy cannot be cancelled and premiums cannot be increased.

The cost of critical illness insurance depends upon:

- Type and range of illnesses covered
- Age and sex of the applicant
- Lump-sum amount of coverage to be purchased

The older the applicant, the higher the cost of coverage. It may sound like this is an argument for buying critical illness coverage at a younger age, but the problem is that most younger people have other priorities in their twenties and thirties: paying down student debt, establishing a household, paying for children's expenses and so on. Furthermore, most younger people do not appreciate the influence of inflation. With an inflation rate at 3%, a policy of $200,000 when purchased at age 25 would need to be increased to $400,000 by age 49 just to maintain the equivalent purchasing power. The cost for most young people would be prohibitive.

It is most likely that the people purchasing critical illness insurance will be in their forties and fifties, when they can afford the cost.

The amount of critical illness coverage that can be purchased ranges from $10,000 to $2 million.

The following table illustrates premium variations at different ages.

Age, Sex and Smoking Status at Purchase of Policy	Amount of Lump-sum Payment (dollars)	Yearly Cost of 10–Year Renewal Premiums Each 10 Years (dollars)		Yearly Cost of Level Premium to Age 75 (dollars)	Riders
Female, non-smoker, age 25	$100,000	0–10 years	$297	$481	Disability waiver, return of premium
		10–20 years	$413		
		20–30 years	$724		
		30–40 years	$1,308		
Female, non-smoker, age 35	$100,000	0–10 years	$423	$806	Disability waiver, return of premium
		10–20 years	$738		
		20–30 years	$1,329		
Female, non-smoker age 55	$100,000	0–10 years	$1,091	$1,559	Disability waiver, return of premium
		10–20 years	$2,393		
Female, smoker, age 55	$100,000	1–10 years	$3,712	$4,058	Disability waiver, return of premium
		10–20 years	$7,452		

Who Should Consider Buying Critical Illness Insurance?

Consider buying critical illness insurance if you:

- Already have disability insurance in force, but have surplus income and want to have a little more protection against the costs of a life-threatening disease
- Are newly self-employed and unable to obtain disability insurance during the transition years
- Are unable to obtain sufficient disability insurance
- Are not in the workforce at all and cannot insure earnings
- Have additional responsibilities such as parents, children or spouse who require caregiving

For these people, critical illness insurance may make sense, depending on individual circumstances. Always contact an insurance professional to obtain quotes from at least three different companies. Review the covered illnesses and assess the value to you of each type of coverage before making a decision.

Tip: CompCorp provides Canadian life insurance policyholders with specified levels of protection against loss of benefits due to the financial failure of a Member Insurance Company. There are limits on coverage depending on the type of insurance. Critical Illness Benefits are guaranteed to a lump-sum maximum of $60,000. If you are considering purchasing more than this maximum coverage, consider splitting the coverage between two or more different insurance companies.

Group Critical Illness Coverage

Some employers offer critical illness insurance as part of their supplementary health or extended health benefits package. Often, the lump-sum payment amount is determined as a percentage of the employee's salary, or it can be a percentage of the employee's life insurance benefit. Because these are part of group plans, the coverage is more restricted than individual plans.

Tip: If an employee has life insurance, and contracts a terminal illness, then life insurance companies will sometimes agree to pay out some lump-sum benefits instead of waiting for the employee's death to pay out benefits. Critical illness coverage gives more certainty of payout in the event of a serious, terminal illness.

Other Sources of Critical Illness Insurance

Some life insurance companies are combining critical illness policies with life insurance policies. At the time of purchase of a life insurance policy, a percentage (typically between 25% and 75%) of the face value of the term life insurance can be designated as critical illness insurance. In the event of covered illness or disability, the life insurance policy will pay out this amount. The balance will be available if death should follow. If the policyholder dies without using the critical illness component, the full amount will be paid out. Expect to see many different variations on this theme over the next few years.

CRITICAL ILLNESS INSURANCE CHECKLIST

✔ What are the defined conditions covered by the critical illness insurance policy?
✔ Is there a waiting period or survival period?
✔ What amount of coverage is available?
✔ Are you within the age range to purchase a critical illness policy (usually 18 to 65)
✔ What are the conditions for the return of premium?
✔ Is the benefit paid out as a lump sum or as a dollar value for medical treatments?

✔ What riders are available?

✔ Can the critical illness insurance policy be combined with disability or life insurance plans?

✔ Until what age can benefits be paid out? To claimant's age 75? Or for life?

Other Factors To Consider

Because critical illness insurance is a relatively new type of insurance in Canada, there is concern that insurance companies may not be able to continue offering guaranteed premiums that cannot be adjusted to reflect cost increases in underwriting claims.

Discussion in the insurance industry is divided over the impact that improved medical diagnostic tools may have on policies. Some feel there will be an increase in the number of illnesses diagnosed, and therefore, in the number of claims. But early detection may also mean that certain illnesses may not become life threatening, which would reduce claims.

As critical illness insurance evolves, some insurance companies have already changed the focus of their benefits to provide a stated dollar value of medical treatments as opposed to a lump-sum settlement. This is of interest to those who want to have access to more expensive medical treatment: with $1 million in coverage, they may be able to get medical care in the United States that is not available in Canada. It is important that people purchasing critical illness coverage be very clear about the type of policy they are purchasing.

LONG TERM CARE INSURANCE

Given the strain on health care facilities for chronic care, many people are anxious to ensure that they will have some discretionary sources of income in the event that they or their loved ones find themselves in a care facility or require care at home. This is where the innovative product, *long term care insurance*, fits into the picture.

Those Canadians who have saved for their retirement may also be asked to pay for some of their own health care in addition to their regular living expenses. Home care has been a political buzzword for several years now—but not much has really been allocated to make it a possibility for many people. The level of care in provincial institutions for people with disabilities and the elderly has been under increasing financial stress. Some young people with disabilities have been forced to live in senior citizen facilities because nothing is available for them in the community.

Studies show that 42% of Canadians are concerned about having to care for elderly parents even as they, the adult children, grow older. About 47% of Canadians are concerned about becoming a burden themselves.

What is Long Term Care Insurance?

Long term care insurance in the Canadian setting is intended to top up provincial health care plans. Each province provides a minimum level of care for people with disabilities and for the elderly. Long term care insurance allows the person with a disability or the elderly person to pay for at-home care in order to avoid being institutionalized. These benefits also give people the option of selecting a more expensive care facility than would otherwise be possible. Residents of a nursing home can use the funds from long term care insurance benefits to obtain extra services that will enhance their lifestyle.

As with critical illness insurance, the willingness of an insurance company to insure you depends upon the company's research into your health. Your family health history or pre-existing conditions may mean that you are not a desirable risk for the insurance company. There may be extra premium costs, or you may simply be declined coverage.

How Does Long Term Care Insurance Work?

Rather than a fixed lump-sum amount, the applicant applies to the insurance company for coverage of a certain dollar amount per day, typically from $50 to $300 per day.

Applicants usually range in age from 30 years to 80 years. There are different types of plans offered by different companies.

In many cases, medical tests are not required. But some people may not even be considered for long term care insurance based on their family medical history. For example, people who have Alzheimer's or dementia, muscular dystrophy, Parkinson's disease, stroke, multiple sclerosis, or who have received Canada Pension Plan disability benefits or benefits from a long term disability plan would not be considered for coverage.

Once a person has been accepted for long term care insurance, claims can be made only if a physician certifies that the person is either unable to perform two or more activities of daily living (for example, eating, bathing, dressing, toileting, transferring position), or has a cognitive impairment (an inability to think, reason, perceive or remember), which includes such conditions as Alzheimer's disease.

If the claim is accepted, and the waiting period has passed, then the daily benefit is paid out for life or for a specific period of time such as 5 years, depending on the coverage chosen. Benefit payments may be made monthly, semi-annually or annually.

What is Covered by Long Term Care insurance?

Some policies pay the benefit for care in a facility (such as a nursing or retirement home) or for the reimbursement of services provided by licensed health care agencies to provide home care. Such services include the following:

• Housekeeping

- Home maintenance
- In-home nursing
- Occupational therapy
- Respiratory therapy
- Adult day care
- Respite care
- Nursing home care, over and beyond provincial care levels
- Provision of certain medical equipment

Other policies will pay out the daily amount to the policyholder once a physician's diagnosis is received *regardless* of how the money is to be spent. This gives total control to the policyholder to hire care providers and services. It allows for the use of non-licensed caregivers, taxis for transportation, or paying a neighbour to provide some homemaking tasks. These policies are generally more expensive than those requiring the use of licensed practitioners. Keep in mind that the care level provided by licensed and trained caregivers may be superior, although sometimes more expensive, than untrained help.

Types of Long Term Care Insurance Plans

There are several different types of long term care insurance plans.

The main types of policies are as follows:

- *Reimbursement plans* or proof-of-service plans in which payment is based on receipts submitted for care (with any surplus being carried forward).
- *Indemnity plans* that require proof from the policyholder that the care or service was provided, but receipts are not required. Excess funds are paid out in full up to the maximum per month under the plan.
- *Income-based plans* that pay a fixed, contractual amount regardless of whether expenses reach the maximum under the plan. No proof of service is

required. This type of plan allows the policyholder to choose who will provide needed services.

Some plans provide for an *annuity* purchase program that allows the individual to pay for premiums through an annuity income stream. The annuity payments (from *a term certain annuity*) pay the insurance premiums as well as the tax on the part of the annuity that is taxable. This is a useful option for those people who wish to prepay parents' long term care coverage. But it is not used much because interest rates are currently low, and therefore, annuity payouts are also low. Furthermore, most policies have *waiver of premium* option in force once payouts begin. With an annuity, the client could be stuck with the annuity, but with nothing to fund with it, (because the long term care insurance will be paid out with no further premiums to pay) and still have tax payable on the annuity.

The long term care insurance contract is usually *guaranteed renewable, with increasing premiums.* This means that the premiums remain the same for a specified period of time such as 10 years. After that time, the issuing company guarantees that the policyholder is able to renew coverage for an additional period of time, but at an increased premium. Ideally, the policy should provide a maximum premium amount on renewal.

Some policies have a limited premium-payment period, much like paid-up life insurance. The payment period, for example, can be for 10, 15 or 20 years. At the end of that time, the policy is paid for and no further premiums are required for that level of coverage.

Some policies limit the length of time benefits are paid, for example, 2 years or 5 years.

Policy Riders

Additional features or riders can be added to the policy, which will increase the premiums, of course. Such riders may include the following:

Respite care

A provision for respite care for caregivers up to a certain number of days per year may be added to the policy. This enables caregivers to go on vacation or otherwise have time free from their caregiving role.

Waiver of premium

The waiver of premium option means that if the policyholder becomes disabled (or the owner of the policy dies or becomes disabled, if the owner is someone other than the policyholder) there would be no premiums payable, but the policy coverage would continue.

Spousal coverage

Coverage for the spouse of an insured person can be added to some policies at a discounted rate.

Return of premium

The return of premium rider provides that, if death occurs before a certain age and the policy has been in force for a minimum number of years, then a percentage of premiums paid to the date of death (minus any claims made) will be refunded to the surviving spouse or to the deceased's estate. As with critical illness and disability insurance, the cost for this rider can be high.

Cost of living protection

The cost of living adjustment (COLA) provides inflation protection on the policy. (For more information on cost of living protection riders, see Chapter 4, "Disability Insurance".)

Future purchase option

The future purchase option allows for the purchase of additional coverage up to a certain amount without a medical.

What is the Cost of Long Term Care insurance?

The cost of long term care insurance depends upon the age of the applicant and the amount of coverage required. It also depends on the options selected. It is a complex form of insurance because there are many choices to be made. For example, a policy for a male non-smoker age 55 for 2-year coverage of $100 per day for home care and for $100 per day of lifetime facility care with a cost-of-living increase at the time of claim costs $184.35 per month. Premiums are payable for 20 years for a total cost of $40,966. The potential benefit is $36,400 per year for life. The rate is guaranteed for the first 5 years, with potential increases capped.

Some Considerations with Long Term Care Insurance

If the recipient of the long term care services cannot choose or hire his or her own caregivers under the policy, then the care is provided through licensed home care agencies that hire the caregivers. The recipient therefore has no control over the hiring, suitability testing, or firing of these caregivers. In many jurisdictions, there is inadequate supervision of both the facilities and the caregivers by government. Family members and friends often must become advocates for the person receiving care if the care is deficient.

In several cultures, care of the family member with a disability or an elderly family member is left to other family members. In many instances, any payment to the caregiver is an under-the-table transaction, and may not reflect any excellence in the care provided.

Who Should Consider Buying Long Term Care Insurance?

People in the following circumstances may want to consider buying long term care insurance:
- Those who already have disability insurance in place, but who want to augment their coverage in the event of a severe disability requiring care, or to prepare for possible needs as they age.
- Single people with no family members on whom they could rely for care in the event of disability or frailty in old age.
- People with a family history that shows the need for long term care
- Homemakers and others who are not able to purchase disability insurance.

What to Look For in Long Term Care Insurance

It is important to compare different policies and think about different options. For example, the right to hire (or have your spouse or children hire on your behalf) your own caregiver has pros and cons. On the plus side, you, or your representative, has the authority to control who provides your care. On the negative side, children may decide to put in place lower-cost care to save a few dollars to build up their inheritance. Some long term care policies allow payment only to people working for licensed private healthcare providers. Under these policies, the premium rates are capped and are lower than those in policies that allow the claimant the freedom to choose caregivers.

For those who live in major urban centres, where there is a good choice of licensed caregivers, a policy requiring licensed providers may be the best option. The more liberal benefit may be suitable for those in remote areas, where licensed caregivers are scarce or non-existent, so that hiring the neighbour who is unemployed is the only option.

It is important to look at the various provisions of the policy versus the cost. Remember that if you are purchasing coverage 20 years ahead of when you expect to need it, inflation over that time will have reduced the value of the amount you purchased, possibly quite substantially.

Make sure that you understand the ramifications of purchasing a policy that ends before age 90. Long term care is most often needed in the last few years of life. A policy that expires at age 75, when as a female, your life expectancy is currently expected to be age 86, probably makes little sense.

Avoid paying extra premiums for return of premium guarantee on long term care insurance. It is better to purchase more coverage or a cost-of-living rider.

Planning Ideas for Long Term Care Insurance

Because long term care insurance is a relatively new type of insurance, the insurance companies are developing new and innovative products.

One product expected soon would offer the option to convert an existing disability insurance policy at age 65 into a long term care plan. Of course, premiums would be at current rates at the time of conversion, but with the possibility that the long term care policy would not require a medical or questionnaire. This is not available at time of writing.

If you have an existing life insurance policy or are approaching age 65 when most disability insurance stops, consider *reallocating* the premium dollars to long term care insurance when life or disability insurance is no longer needed. Generally, you no longer need life or disability insurance once your children are grown, you have no debts, and you have reached age 65. This strategy also works well when there is permanent life insurance (such as *whole life*), which may not really be needed. The life insurance premiums can be redirected to long term care insurance and any accumulated value in the life insurance policy can be used to pay premiums or for other purposes.

Tip: CompCorp provides Canadian life insurance policyholders with specified levels of protection against loss of benefits due to the financial failure of a Member Insurance Company. There are limits on coverage depending on the type of insurance. Long term Care insurance benefits are guaranteed to a maximum of $2,000 per month. If you are considering purchasing more than this maximum coverage, consider splitting the coverage between two different insurance companies.

Group Long Term Care Insurance

Group extended health plans and other employee benefit plans are starting to offer long term care insurance as an option. (See Chapter 5, "Employee Benefit and Individual Plans.") This is being offered more and more to retirees as a supplementary option to extended health plans. Of course, there is a price to pay and, as with all plans, it is important to look at how long the coverage lasts and what it covers before signing on. Individuals must also look at whether they can afford the additional premiums. As with most group insurance, the cost is usually cheaper than individual plans because of a larger number of people to share the risk.

LONG TERM CARE INSURANCE CHECKLIST

✔ What is the definition that triggers payment of benefits? For example, an inability to perform two or more of activities of daily living, which are stated in the policy, or mental incapacity that might result in harm coming to the individual if care is not provided.

✔ What type of plan is it: reimbursement plan, indemnity plan, fixed income plan?

✔ What is the benefit amount?

✔ Will coverage include home care and facility care?

✔ What is the waiting period: 30, 90, 180 days?

✔ How long will benefits last: 1 year, 3 years, 5 years or, life?

✔ How long will premiums have to be paid: monthly, for a limited time?

✔ Does the policyholder have control over who provides care? Or are caregivers provided through service contracted by the insurance company?

✔ Is there flexibility as to the purposes for which benefit payments can be used?

✔ Is there a return of premium feature? What are the conditions?

✔ What riders are available?

✔ What are the exclusions on the policy?

COMPARISON OF DISABILITY INSURANCE WITH CRITICAL ILLNESS AND LONG TERM CARE INSURANCE

	Disability Insurance	Critical Illness Insurance	Long Term Care Insurance
Eligible Policyholders	Those earning an income from employment or self-employment	Anyone who has been accepted on health grounds up to age maximum	Anyone who pays premium for stated amount of coverage and is within age range for coverage
Purpose of Coverage	To replace earned income	To pay out one-time lump sum if covered ailment is life threatening	To pay for care in a nursing home or to provide at home care when ability to perform 2 or more activities of daily living is impaired

	Disability Insurance	Critical Illness Insurance	Long term Care Insurance
Criteria for Coverage	Must earn income from some type of employment; Must meet health tests; Age/sex also determinants of coverage	No earnings test; Must meet health tests; Age/sex also determinants of coverage	Must be within age range for policy to start; must pay premiums; must meet health criteria of issuer
Diagnosis of Ailment Required for Payout	Unless client cannot work, no payment is made	If covered ailment is life threatening, then diagnosis means payout	Pays out if policyholder unable to perform at least 2 basic tasks of daily living
Frequency of Benefit Paid Out	Monthly, according to policy terms	One-time, lump-sum payout; or treatment up to stated amount	May be weekly, monthly for specified period or for life
Amount of Benefit Paid Out	Depends on pre-disability income; maximum benefit is stated in contract. Maybe reduced by CPP disability or worker's compensation payments	Depends upon amount of lump-sum coverage selected under policy	Depends upon amount, frequency and duration of coverage selected

SOURCES OF INFORMATION

The Insurance Journal – www.insurance-journal.ca/archives
Year 2000 figures quoted from "The Insurance Journal", Vol. 5, #6

The Canadian Life and Health Insurance Association (CLHIA) has a Consumer Assistance Centre at 1-800-268-8099; in Toronto the number is 416-777-2344; Web site at www.clhia.ca.

CompCorp for information on guaranteed insurance coverage:
Contact the Consumer Assistance Centre at 1-800-268-8099 toll free or 416-777-2344
E-mail CompCorp at: info@compcorp.ca
CompCorp Web site www.compcorp.ca

Web sites of major life insurance companies in Canada that carry disability, critical illness or long term care insurance products.

CHAPTER 7

FEDERAL GOVERNMENT PROGRAMS

CANADA PENSION PLAN DISABILITY BENEFITS

Disability benefits from the Canada Pension Plan (CPP) first became available in 1970. Since then, there have been a number of revisions to the rules and regulations, most recently in 1997. Currently, about 60% of CPP disability applications are denied, and it is likely that this percentage will increase as a result of the latest changes in guidelines.

However, a subcommittee of the federal government is currently reviewing submissions regarding CPP disability benefits and pressure is building for relaxing the rules for CPP disability claimants. Most CPP disability benefit beneficiaries are between the ages of 50 and 64, with about 43% under the age of 55. About 88% of CPP disability beneficiaries suffer from mobility impairments. In 2000, some 283,508 Canadians were receiving CPP disability benefits.

Both CPP and QPP in Quebec, in addition to providing retirement benefits to working Canadians, provide disability benefits to working Canadians who are unable to work due to a *severe and prolonged disability*. The cost of providing both retirement and disability benefits is covered by contributions to CPP made by employers and employees. The funds are then invested to cover the cost of pensions and claims.

All workers who earn more than $3,500 per year contribute to CPP at a percentage rate based on their Year's Maximum Pensionable Earnings (YMPE). The YMPE changes annually and is set by the federal government. In 2003, it is $39,900. Currently, the contribution rate is rising to 10% of YMPE, so that the maximum dollar contribution to CPP will be approximately $3,600 per year and indexed each year. Employees contribute one half of the required annual amount, employers the remaining half. People who are self-employed contribute both halves of the amount. Only employed and self-employed people can contribute to CPP—no one can make voluntary CPP contributions.

The purpose of CPP disability benefits is to provide disabled Canadian workers with a *base level* of income support. It was never intended to be the major source of disability income coverage. Indeed, the assumption was that the coverage would be equal to no more than 25% of the average industrial wage or 25% of the earnings on which the contributor paid into the plan, whichever is lower. The coverage has the following characteristics:

- *Universal*: All workers who have contributed to the plan are eligible to apply for benefits in the event of disability.
- *Fully indexed*: The amount of the benefit increases each year to reflect inflation.
- *Portable*: Workers can move from employer to employer and province to province as employees or employers. And they can start their own businesses and still be covered by CPP benefits. Note that benefits under QPP are somewhat different and will be discussed later in this chapter.
- A *Defined Benefit* program: All payments are based on a fixed percentage of employment earnings up to the average wage and averaged out over the claimant's working life.

Although CPP pensions and disability benefits are important to both men and women in Canada, they are critically important for women because fewer women workers are protected under employer-sponsored retirement or disability protection programs.

There are certain advantages to CPP disability benefits that are not available through most other income replacement programs. Coverage is extended to all contributors:

- Regardless of the type of work they do
- Whether they are self-employed or employees

- Regardless of previous medical history
- Until recovery from the disability, retirement, or death, whichever occurs first

CPP disability benefits are not permanent, and there is no provision for partial benefits to be paid. There are no supplemental payments for medical equipment or health-related services.

How the CPP Benefit System Works

To receive CPP Disability benefits, a claimant must
- Suffer a *severe and prolonged mental or physical disability* that prevents him/her from regularly working in any substantially gainful occupation
- Meet the *minimum contributory requirements* as set out in regulations

Definition of disability as *severe and prolonged*
CPP uses a rigid definition of disability. CPP disability income is intended to provide a base level of income for people who are *permanently and totally disabled and unable to work in any occupation.*

CPP defines a *severe* disability as one that makes a person *incapable of regularly pursuing any substantially gainful occupation.*

This definition of *severe* has been interpreted both narrowly and widely in different cases. In some situations, in addition to the claimant's inability to work, such real-life circumstances as the claimant's age, education level and language proficiency are taken into account.

CPP defines a *prolonged* disability as one that is likely to be *long, continued and of indefinite duration or is likely to result in death.* For example, a truck driver who has a broken leg that will keep him off work for 6 months will not be eligible to receive a CPP disability benefit.

In many cases, the age of the claimant may determine whether the definition of severe and prolonged is interpreted broadly or narrowly. An older claimant close to retirement age may be able to obtain CPP disability benefits, whereas a younger claimant with the same disability may be denied.

Contributory requirements

To receive benefits, workers must have

- Paid into CPP for 4 out of the last 6 years, with a minimum of 4 contribution years. Contributions are made on earned income between $3,500 and the Yearly Maximum Pensionable Earnings (YMPE) of $39,900 in 2003.
- Contributed on earnings equal to 10% of the YMPE; thus the minimum contributory income to collect CPP disability benefits required in 2003 was $3,990.
- Applied for benefits. Workers may apply as late applicants if they were disabled for more than 15 months before they made their application. Retroactive benefits may therefore be paid for up to 15 months before the date of application.

There are circumstances in which a person with a disability may still qualify for CPP disability benefits even though they have not technically contributed for the required number of years. You may still receive benefits if one of these conditions applies:

- If you can claim the *child-raising dropout provision* (see below)
- If you received CPP credits from a spouse as the result of separation or divorce
- If you worked in another country and contributed to its social security plan and that country has an agreement with Canada for benefit entitlements
- If you were previously receiving CPP disability benefits that stopped when you returned to work, but the disability has recurred, as long as required

contributions have been made after you returned to work. In this case, the requirement of contributions to CPP in 4 out of the last 6 years may be waived.

- If you were medically unable to apply and now no longer meet the 4 out of 6 years contribution requirement
- If there was a delay in applying (if the application had been made immediately upon disability, you would have qualified; however, now you do not qualify.)

Benefit Calculations

Once it has been determined that you meet the contributory requirements and definition of disability, there are other calculations that CPP performs to determine the *earnings related component* of the disability benefit. There are several parts to this calculation.

- CPP does not include the lowest 15% of your contributory earnings years. This means that there is a higher average calculated on your earned income and therefore a higher amount of potential benefit.
- CPP also factors in the *child-raising dropout provision* that allows a parent to discount years of lower earnings or no earnings while they were raising children under the age of 7. There is no limit to the number of years that may be claimed under this provision since it depends upon the number of children you have and whether you were away from the workforce during their early years (up to each child's age 7). If you earned little or no income during each of those years, then those low-income years will be not be counted when calculating the amount of benefit and contributory years.

- Contributions to both QPP and CPP are combined for claimants who may have worked in both Quebec and another province. Only one application is required.

Calculating contributory requirements and qualifying provisions for CPP (or QPP) is complex. Visit a local office, go to the Web site, phone, write, or fax, Human Resources Development Canada (HRDC), the government department that administers the Canada Pension Plan, in order to get help. (See details at the end of the chapter.)

Amount of Canada Pension Plan Disability Benefit

There are two parts to disability payments under CPP.

Part I is the *flat rate component*, which is payable to all beneficiaries. For 2003, it was $370.32 per month.

Part II is the *earnings-related component*. It is equal to 75% of the retirement pension that the contributor would have received at age 65 to a maximum amount ($600.94 per month in 2003).

The combined maximum benefit for each year is stated on the CPP Web site. For 2003, it was $971.26 per month or $11,655.12 per year. The average monthly benefit actually paid to claimants in October, 2002, was $718.90.

People who receive a CPP *survivor's retirement pension* may also be entitled to a disability benefit in their own right, if they meet the requirements and if they have contributed to CPP based on their own earnings. (A CPP survivor's pension is one that is paid to the widow or widower of a CPP contributor.) However, the total amount of the combined survivor's and disability benefit cannot exceed the maximum disability benefit available in the year in which the person becomes eligible for the second CPP benefit. The average combined survivor's and disability benefit in October 2002 was $864.

There is also a *child benefit* under the CPP disability plan. It is paid as a flat rate, which was $186.71 per month in 2003. It is *not* granted automatically. You must apply for it on behalf of the qualified child. The child must be under age 18 or between ages 18 and 25 and in full-time attendance at a recognized school or university. Children over the age of 18 must apply on their own behalf and supply proof of full-time attendance at a school or university. Children may receive more than one benefit amount if both parents are disabled or have died.

Integration of CPP with other Benefits

CPP is usually the *first payor* for disability claims. This means that other plans are the *second payors*, which will *top up* the amount received by the claimant for CPP disability benefits. Put another way, if you receive disability benefits from another source, in addition to CPP, the amount you receive from the other source is reduced by the amount that you receive from CPP. Examples of second payors are some group disability plans, provincial social security programs for people with disabilities and workers' compensation plans. Individual and private disability insurance plans are not usually reduced by CPP disability payments.

Integration of CPP with Overseas Plans

Immigrants, or Canadians who have been employed in other countries, may have claims for disability payments from the social security programs of those countries. However, the definitions of disability, and therefore the grounds for payment, vary from country to country.

If the person with the disability does not have the mandatory 4 contribution years in Canada, eligibility for plans in other countries where he or she has worked should be investigated. Whether those benefits are integrated will depend on the Social Security treaty between Canada and the other country.

Applying for CPP Disability Benefits

Application kits are available from Human Resources Development Canada (HRDC) at 1-800-277-9914. Here's what you will need:

- The applicant's birth or baptismal certificate
- A birth or baptismal certificate for each child listed on the disability or child-rearing dropout provision application
- The applicant's social insurance card
- Medical reports, hospital discharge summaries or other information about the applicant's disability so that HRDC can assess the disability

Note that photocopies are acceptable but they must be *certified true copies*. A notary or other qualified person, as described in the application instructions, can certify copies of the applicant's information.

If a person is incapable of applying him or herself, a representative may apply for him or her. This person does not have to be officially assigned (such as a holder of power of attorney) to make this application. A special form, called the *Declaration of Incapacity—Physicians report (I SP 1800)* will be required.

If the application is approved, the applicant receives a *notice of entitlement* that states:

- The date benefits begin
- The amount of the monthly benefit
- The amount of first payment, including retroactive payments
- Information on the beneficiary's rights and responsibilities

The first payment is normally issued within 30 working days after the applicant receives the notice of entitlement. This is normally 4 months after the onset of the disability. Disability benefits are indexed to inflation, and each January, the amount is adjusted according to the Consumer Price Index.

A T4 slip is issued at the beginning of each year for the previous calendar year, and beneficiaries must declare that income on their tax return for the year. CPP disability income qualifies as *earned income* for RRSP contribution purposes, which means that RRSP contributions can be made based on the amount of CPP disability income received, just as if the income was earned from a regular job.

CPP disability benefits are not available on behalf of deceased applicants unless the application was received before the date of death. In a case where the application was received by HRDC before the applicant's death, a surviving spouse, dependent children or the estate would receive any benefits payable up to the applicant's date of death.

A surviving spouse and dependent children may be eligible for survivor's benefits under the CPP retirement pension.

How Long do CPP Disability Payments Continue?

CPP disability benefits stop under the following circumstances:

- The beneficiary is longer considered disabled under the terms of CPP legislation. According to legislation, if your disability is no longer classified as *severe and prolonged* and you have regained the ability to engage in *substantially gainful occupation*, benefits will stop.
- The beneficiary is age 65, at which time the disability pension is replaced by a retirement pension.
- The beneficiary dies.

The Appeals Process

What happens when an application is denied?
Nurse adjudicators screen the initial application for CPP disability benefits. Claimants who are rejected may appeal the decision.

Why are some CPP disability benefit claims denied?
Applications for CPP disability benefits are denied because
- The claimant has not made enough contributions to the plan
- The disability does not meet the *severe and prolonged* criteria
- The disability began after the applicant's 65th birthday

What are some grounds for appeal?
You may appeal the decision if
- You disagree with the amount of the benefit to be paid
- The date when the disability began is in dispute
- The calculation of the date of the commencement of benefit payments is in dispute

What are the stages of appeals?

Reconsideration or Administrative Review
The first level of appeal is called a *reconsideration* or *administrative review*. It is made within HRDC, the department of the federal government that oversees CPP applications, by an adjudicator who was not involved in the initial assessment of the case. You must request a reconsideration within 90 days of when you receive the rejection of your initial claim. New evidence, if any, to prove your case can be introduced at this time. Up-to-date medical reports and assessments, and evidence of earlier onset of the disability are examples of new evidence. Typically, each year there are about 20,000

appeals for this level of adjudication, but about 72% of these appeals are denied.

Level 82 Appeals

The next level of appeal is to the Office of the Commissioner of Review Tribunals (OCRT). All parties may be represented by an advocate or a lawyer if they wish. The three members on the Tribunal are chosen from a pool of several hundred members of the Review Tribunal. The chair must be a lawyer and one of the other members must be qualified to practice medicine or a related profession. The third member is a member of the public. The hearing is closed to the public.

Pension Appeals Board

At this final level of appeal, the Board that hears the appeal is made up of three retired judges. To get an appeal heard by this Board, you must apply and get permission to appeal. If permission to appeal is not granted, the decision of the Tribunal is final. This Board hearing is open to the public.

Many group disability insurance companies integrate their benefits with CPP, that is, they reduce the amount of the benefit you receive by the amount that you are able to get from CPP. As such, most insurance companies will *require* that disabled claimants apply for CPP disability and follow the appeals process to the limit, regardless of the likelihood of success. This probably accounts for a large number of appeals denied at the first level.

Calculating Retirement Benefits for Disabled Beneficiaries

If the usual rules for calculating the amount of CPP retirement benefits were used, a person collecting CPP disability benefits would be at a disadvantage by having a significantly lower level of retirement benefit at age 65. This is because they would have had a shorter contribution period compared with people who have had a standard working career ending at age 65. Therefore, years during which a contributor was receiving CPP disability benefits are excluded from the calculation of the retirement benefit that begins when the disability benefit ends at age 65. This means that people who are totally disabled and receiving CPP benefits are not financially penalized during their retirement years because of their disability. CPP retirement pension calculations are based on the Yearly Maximum Pensionable Earnings *at the time of disability*, regardless of when this occurred, plus indexation of benefits.

Quebec Pension Plan

Although it is similar in most respects to the Canada Pension Plan, there are some important differences in the Quebec Pension Plan.

- Quebec applicants will be assessed retroactively for only a period of up to 1 year before they made the application, and benefits are payable retro-actively for only 8 months.
- Quebec generally applies stricter eligibility criteria and adjudication to applicants under the age of 60, but this is partially offset by a more liberal treatment in recognizing difficulties older workers may face returning to their previous occupations.
- QPP disability benefits beneficiaries appear to be older as a group than those for CPP.
- QPP has a smaller group of beneficiaries who have mental or emotional disorders or who have repetitive strain injuries.
- QPP does reassessments when the medical personnel deem it appropriate; CPP does them when the beneficiary returns to work, or as a result of third party information, or when there has been a scheduled reassessment.
- QPP is more integrated with other forms of prov-incial assistance such as workers' compensation

and provincial disability benefits, as well as the Quebec auto insurance plan. As a result, claimants may receive payments *either* under workers' compensation or QPP, but not both.

In addition, the rules and regulations regarding QPP Pension Credit Splitting on divorce or separation differ from the CPP rules. Couples who have contributed only to QPP (i.e., neither spouse has ever worked outside Quebec) should therefore contact La Regie des rentes du Quebec for information.

Returning to Work

If you are receiving CPP disability benefits and you return to work, you need to inform HRDC once you earn $3,800. If you are able to work only periodically, you may be able to earn more than $3,800 in the year.

Once a beneficiary has returned to work, there is normally a 3-month trial period before the benefits are cancelled. If the attempt to return to work is unsuccessful, benefits continue. If, during the following 5 years, you become disabled again due to the same medical problems, you may be able to use the *Fast Track* reapplication process.

Self-employed CPP disability pension beneficiaries are required to inform HRDC once they have gross income of $3,800 in a year. Their income is then monitored on a monthly basis and benefits will continue to be paid until they have had monthly income in excess of $778 per month, after their business expenses have been paid, for 4 months.

People receiving CPP disability benefits are allowed to do volunteer work, attend school or retraining programs without reporting to HRDC as long as they remain disabled. This may not be the case with many employer-sponsored disability plans.

The CPP Vocational Rehabilitation Program

The CPP Vocational Rehabilitation Program is designed to help people with severe and prolonged disabilities return to employment. This is an individualized program that provides comprehensive vocational rehabilitation services through private businesses across Canada. To be accepted into the program, you must:

- Be medically stable
- Be motivated and willing to participate
- Be referred by a doctor as a suitable candidate
- Be a Canadian resident
- Be receiving CPP disability benefits
- Be likely to return to work with the help received from a vocational rehabilitation program

Upon completion of the program, participants have a 3-month job search period. This search period may be extended to 1 year in exceptional circumstances. There is also a 3-month work-trial provision. CPP benefits stop once people show that they have regained their capacity to work.

Some Pitfalls to Avoid:

- Some employer group plan sponsors, or disability payors may actively encourage those receiving disability benefits to take *early retirement options*. This could be a costly mistake. If you decide to take your CPP retirement benefits before you turn 65, the amount you receive is reduced by half of 1% per month for each month that you are under the age of 65. This is a 30% reduction if you take it at age 60. The maximum CPP retirement benefit at age 60 (in 2003) was about $6,730 per year. But the maximum annual CPP disability benefit is $11,655. This is a significant difference in income! Additionally, if you take the CPP retirement benefit, you also lose the child benefit for any children attending school or university.

- Some advisors tell potential CPP disability claimants not to apply for the CPP benefit. They give two reasons for this:
  - First, the group disability plan payments will be reduced by the amount paid by CPP if the plan is integrated; therefore the claimant should not bother to apply for CPP disability unless required to do so by the group disability insurance company. However, if more than 15 months elapses before the insurance company requires you to make a CPP disability claim (8 months in Quebec), then the CPP retirement pension you will be entitled to at age 65 may be lower.
  - Secondly, if there is a *tort liability claim*, in other words, if you can sue (see Chapter 12, "When Can you Sue"), the courts may count all sources of income (including CPP disability payments) when assessing your income, which could reduce the amount of the settlement you receive. However, your CPP retirement pension will be higher if you take CPP disability benefits sooner rather than later, so you have to weigh your options. A professional advisor who is familiar with CPP issues should evaluate these possibilities.
- Canada Pension Plan credits can be split between the spouses in the event of divorce, but the amount of credit you get is only for the duration of the marriage or common law relationship.
- Since the disabling event may be extremely severe and the prognosis not particularly good, it is important to remember that CPP disability no longer pays benefits to estates if the person with the disability dies. Once the person has survived beyond 4 months, CPP disability payments will be made until age 65, recovery or death whichever

occurs first. Therefore, it is important to apply for disability benefits as soon as possible after the disabling event.

- Canadians who are between ages 60 and 65 and who have stopped working and think they may qualify for a disability benefit should apply for both the retirement and disability pension. The amount of the disability benefit is higher but takes longer to process. If the retirement benefit is received first and the disability application is approved later, Canada Pension Plan will make the necessary adjustments.

The important point to remember with Canada Pension Plan or Quebec Pension Plan disability benefits is this: Get help in applying—it is complex. But be sure to apply! Government departments and agencies try to explain things simply, but "legalese" creeps in. Do not be deterred from making an application or appealing when necessary.

EMPLOYMENT INSURANCE SICKNESS BENEFITS

All working Canadians, other than those who are self-employed or small business owners, contribute to Employment Insurance (EI) and are entitled to benefits under the *sickness benefits* program as long as they meet all of the following eligibility criteria.

- You must have accumulated at least 600 *insured hours* in the last 52 weeks or since you last claimed for EI benefits.
- Your *regular weekly earnings* have decreased by at least 40% as a result of the sickness.
- You are unable to work because of *sickness, injury,* or *quarantine.*
- You can prove that you are not only unable to work, but that except for the sickness, you would otherwise be available for work.

Benefits are paid to Canadians living in Canada who qualify for EI sickness coverage. Those who qualify for benefits can collect them *outside* Canada only in particular circumstances: if they are going to another country *to receive medical treatment not readily or immediately available in Canada at an accredited hospital, medical clinic or similar facility.* Someone who goes to Florida in February to recuperate from a sickness is not entitled to receive benefits. (Parental and maternity benefits can be collected while the claimant is out of Canada, but this does not apply to sickness benefits.)

How Much is the EI Benefit?

The basic benefit is 55% of your average insured earnings up to a maximum of $413 per week (in 2002). A family with less than $25,921 in income, who has children and receives the child tax benefit, is entitled to the *family supplement.*

For example:

- If your family net income is below $20,921 you will receive the full family supplement.
- If your family net income is $20,000 and you have three children aged 6, 8, and 10, you could receive $86.10 per week plus $4.15 extra supplement because you have a child under 7 years old.
- If your family net income is between $20,921 and $25,921, you will receive a partial family supplement.
- If your family net income is $22,000 and you have three children aged 6, 8, and 10, you could receive $68.20 per week plus $3.45 extra supplement because you have a child under 7 years old.

No family supplement will be paid beyond the maximum EI weekly rate of $413. The family supplement is calculated automatically—no additional application is required.

Applying for EI Sickness Benefits

Applicants must apply either on-line at www.hrdc.gc.ca or in person at their local Human Resources Development Canada (HRDC) office. Applicants need to provide the following:
- Social Insurance Number
- Record of employment for all jobs worked in the previous 52 weeks and details of the most recent employment
- Personal identification such as driver's licence, birth certificate, passport
- Banking information for direct deposit of benefit payments
- Medical certificate stating how long the sickness is expected to last

The waiting period is 2 weeks from the beginning of the claim, with benefit payments starting within 28 days of the start date of the claim. This 2-week waiting period may be waived if the applicant has received paid sick leave from the employer or has received group insurance payments, for at least 2 weeks. In such situations, the employee is considered to have met the 2-week waiting period requirement for EI sickness benefits.

EI Sickness Benefits can last for a maximum of 15 weeks. However, those who also qualify for maternity and parental benefits can combine these benefits with sickness benefits so that the benefit period lasts for 65 weeks as a combined maximum benefit. Note that this depends upon special circumstances that would be worked out through HRDC.

The claimant must complete a report every 2 weeks that is submitted by telephone or by mail.

What affects the amount of EI benefits?

If you receive income from any of the following sources, then your EI payments will be reduced dollar for dollar of income received from these sources:

- Income from employment, including wages and commissions
- Compensation payments from an accident or work-related illness, such as workers' compensation payments
- Income from group insurance, sickness, or loss-of-income plans
- Accident compensation for income replacement from motor vehicle accident claims
- Retirement income from pensions

If you receive income from any of the following sources, then your EI payments *will not* be reduced.

- CPP and QPP disability pensions
- Workers' compensation payments from a permanent settlement
- Insurance benefits under a private plan for sickness benefits
- A private sickness or disability wage-loss replacement plan
- Retroactive pay increases

SOURCES OF INFORMATION

The Canada Pension Plan Disability Benefit, Sherri Torjman. 2002. Prepared for the Office of the Commissioner of Review Tribunals, Caledon Institute of Social Policy

Caledon Institute for Social Policy www.caledoninst.org or telephone 1-613-729-3340

Information Guide on Canada Pension Plan Disability Benefits. Human Resources Development Canada, 1999

Human Resources Development Canada

For more information on Canada Pension Plan benefits and Employment Insurance benefits, go to the HRDC Web site www.hrdc.gc.ca

Tel: 1-800-277-9914 (Press 0 to reach an operator quickly!) TDD/TTY 1-800-255-4786, fax: (819) 953-7260.

Mailing address:

Enquiries Centre,

Human Resources Development Canada,
Hull, Quebec, K1A 0J9

In Quebec, La Regie des rentes de Quebec www.rrq.gouv.qc.ca
(Note that information on this Web site is in French only.)
Employment Insurance: www.hrdc.gc.ca

CHAPTER 8

PROVINCIAL GOVERNMENT BENEFITS

SOCIAL ASSISTANCE PROGRAMS

Social assistance programs, which provide minimum income support and health benefits for people with disabilities, are different from welfare programs offered to other provincial residents. On the surface, they are similar; but there are important differences. Welfare programs are *income-tested* programs: if you have an income that is under a minimum level, you qualify for welfare assistance. Social assistance programs for people with disabilities are granted if the person qualifies for payment based on a number of factors, not just income.

Although it is not practical to explain each provincial social assistance program here, the outline of Ontario's plan shows the major areas of coverage.

In all provinces, these programs are in a constant state of flux. Although every effort has been made to be as up-to-date as possible, you must check with your provincial government agency. These programs are designed to offer support until age 65, at which point Old Age Security, CPP/QPP, and other support systems take over. The following information is for Ontario, although other provinces have similar programs.

Ontario Disability Support Program

The Ontario Disability Support Program (ODSP) provides financial assistance to people with disabilities who are

- Over the age of 18, and
- have had *a substantial physical or mental impairment that is continuous or recurrent*, and

137

- the impairment is *expected to last 1 year or more.*

People eligible for Canada Pension Plan (CPP) disability benefits very likely also qualify for at least partial ODSP benefits, assuming their income is low enough. Someone not eligible for CPP disability benefits may, however, qualify for ODSP, assuming they meet the income and asset tests.

Financial qualifications

There are limits to the amount of money or *assets* you can have and still be eligible for ODSP.

- A single person may have no more than $5,000 total in cash, RRSPs, and cash value of life insurance policies.
- A couple (including a common-law spouse or same-sex partner) may have no more than $7,500 total in cash, RRSPs, or cash value of life insurance policies.
- A couple with children may have no more than $7,500 as above, *plus* $500 for each child.

The maximum payment from ODSP is $930 per month for a single person and $1,417 for a family of two. In Ontario, there has been no increase in ODSP benefits since 1997. Be aware that the ODSP benefit is reduced by income from many sources including, pension income (e.g., Canada Pension); gifts, inheritances, student loans, and support payments from an ex-spouse.

Definition of assets

Instead of defining what *is* included as an asset, ODSP specifically defines what is *not included* as an asset. The following is a partial list of items *not included as assets.* Note that for ODSP's purposes, you and your family become a *benefit unit.*

What is NOT included as an asset

- Necessities of living such as furniture, clothing and household effects. Valuable collectables such as stamps, coin collections and antiques are considered to be assets, although antiques, such as furniture, necessary for personal use, are not considered to be assets.

- A principal residence, (or the proceeds from the sale of a principal residence), is not considered an asset, provided the funds are used for the purchase of another principal residence within 12 months.

- An interest in a second property is exempt if it is considered "necessary for the health or well-being of a member of the benefit unit". Otherwise it will likely be considered an asset.

- The value of one motor vehicle owned by a member of the benefit unit is exempt, and there is no limit to the value of this vehicle. A second vehicle may be exempt if it is required to permit a dependent of the applicant to maintain employment outside the home, but the value of this second vehicle is limited to $15,000.

- Trust funds may be exempt if they are inheritances or proceeds of a life insurance policy placed in trust for the benefit of that person *and have a limit* of $100,000, including reinvested interest and dividends. This includes the cash surrender value of a whole life insurance policy. In other words, the combined trust and life insurance cash surrender value may not exceed $100,000. The value over $100,000 is considered an asset.

- Awards for pain and suffering and expenses are exempt. Up to $100,000 received as a monetary award for pain and suffering, as well as for expenses actually and reasonably incurred as a result of injury to, or death of a member of the benefit unit are not considered assets. Payments under the Workers' Compensation Act and

Workplace Safety and Insurance Act are excluded as assets because they are not considered compensation for pain and suffering.

- Prepaid funerals are exempt.
- Student loans, grants, awards or bursaries are exempt as an asset provided the recipient is in attendance in the program for which the funds were paid. (Caution! See the next section.)
- Business assets up to a value of $20,000 and tools of the trade are also exempt as assets.
- Capital in locked-in RRSPs is not considered to be an asset. (A locked-in RRSP or locked-in retirement account [LIRA] is made up of money transferred from a pension plan into a special type of RRSP. The rules governing these locked-in plans differ significantly from RRSPs, and typically these funds may not be accessed until you are 55 or older. At that point, the funds must be used to generate an income stream.) There may be a significant penalty for taking *income* from the locked-in plan at age 55. But ODSP will require that you do so—and income received from such a locked-in account will be deducted dollar for dollar from benefits payable under ODSP, whether the income is received as an annuity or LIF (Life Income Fund, which comes from a locked-in account when it is converted to an income stream). In other words the locked in RRSP is not an asset, *but* you are required to take income from it at a certain point and then it becomes a source of income! The same thing applies with pensions. A pension plan that allows an early pension payout may not be advantageous to take, but ODSP will require that you do so at the earliest date. The problem with this is that it impacts on your long term financial security during your retirement years.
- Loans for the purchase of exempt assets such as motor vehicles and a principal residence are

exempted both as income and assets, as are loans for the payment of first and last month's rent.

ODSP considers regular RRSPs as assets

If these funds can be accessed by the person with a disability, he or she will be required to do so. (Therefore if an applicant has $20,000 in an RRSP, they will be required to use at least $15,000 of it before they will be eligible for ODSP since there is a $5,000 exemption.)

The ODSP and Henson Trusts (Absolute Discretionary Trusts)

Concerned parents often want to provide additional funds for their disabled children (especially as these children become adults) without causing their adult children to lose their ODSP benefits. Estate planners devised the Henson Trust which is named after a Guelph, Ontario, family. The provisions of the Henson Trust apply only in Ontario.

These trusts can be set up as an Inter Vivos trust (where the settlor, who endows the trust, and the recipient, are both living), or as a Testamentary trust (where the settlor sets the trust up before death and the trust becomes operational only at the settlor's death). Briefly, the trust is set up so that the adult child is not the only possible beneficiary of the trust. Very often, a charitable foundation is named as the trust beneficiary at the child's death. In other words, the trust has more than one potential beneficiary who receives income at the discretion of the trustees. The child who ultimately benefits from the trust does so at the discretion of the trustees: the child does not have an absolute right to the funds. This means that the Province of Ontario cannot exclude the adult child from ODSP benefits on the grounds that the asset maximum of $100,000 for a trust has been surpassed by assets in the trust. The child does not own the assets in the trust, and therefore, the trust assets, since they do not belong to the child, cannot be counted in any list of the child's assets.

When the trust pays out benefits to the beneficiary with the disability, then those payments are considered income and assets in the hands of the child. This is why the trustees have to carefully monitor the amounts which are paid out to the person with the disability each year. These trusts are especially useful when the amount of capital involved in a potential inheritance is going to be over $100,000 and where trust income might otherwise be over $5,000 per year.

Residents of other provinces should check with a knowledgeable estate lawyer to see if a similar option is available in their province.

What is income?

To further complicate the matter, ODSP may not consider some things as assets, but those same things may be considered to be income.

All applicants for ODSP are expected to pursue and obtain any other financial resources to which they or their dependants may be entitled. For example, this typically includes spousal and child support from an ex-spouse of the person with the disability. If you are not able to obtain the income due to you, ODSP will deduct an amount from your benefit that is equal to the income that should have been available.

Income is defined as monies received in a given month, rather than the month in which it is earned or promised.

Some definitions of income are

* Wages, salaries or any other form of earned income
* Any payments received from an annuity, pension plan or insurance benefit
* All payments received from mortgages held
* Any pension payments from any other country
* Any payments for spousal or child support
* Payments received on sale of an asset unless otherwise exempt

- Interest earned from proceeds of a compensation award regardless of the amount of the award
- Interest or dividends from a life insurance policy that is not otherwise exempt
- A percentage of rental income or lodging income
- Any payments received under the following pieces of legislation:
  — Workplace Safety and Insurance or Workers Compensation Acts
  — Pension Act (Canada)
  — Employment Insurance Act
  — War Veterans Allowance Act
  — Civilian's War Pension and Allowances Act
  — Canada or Quebec Pension Plan
  — Old Age Security and Guaranteed Income Supplement
  — Ontario Guaranteed Annual Income Act
  — National Child Benefit Supplement portion of Canada Child Tax Benefit.

Besides everything that is to be included in income, there are also *exclusions*. Some of these exclusions are as follows:

- Up to $160 per month of net employment or training program earnings for one adult in the unit and $235 (families) plus 25% of the amount above these maximums
- Proceeds from the sale of a principal residence, assuming the funds are used to purchase another principal residence within 12 months
- Refundable tax credits such as the Canada Child Tax Benefit except for the supplement
- Ontario childcare supplement for working families
- Student loans received to pay for student financing. Be aware that the exempt portion of student loans applies only to the portion of the loan that pays for tuition, compulsory fees, books, and necessary instructional supplies, and transportation. *Student loans used for living*

expenses are treated as income. Most students who are or were recipients of ODSP will find themselves with a greatly reduced ODSP benefit or, in most cases, no longer eligible for ODSP. This is significant in that students with disabilities end up with large student loan debt, but their job prospects are considerably lower than those for able-bodied students after graduation.

- The proceeds of compensation (either from an insurance or legal settlement) for pain and suffering up to a maximum of $100,000.
- Donations from a religious, charitable or benevolent organization up to $100,000 for the recipient's lifetime, but these are also combined with the amount for an inheritance, trust and/or insurance policy. Therefore, the total from the three sources cannot exceed $100,000.
- Canada or Quebec Pension Plan death benefits

There are many other exemptions not mentioned here. Most of the information is available on the provincial government Web site.

✗ **Warning:** As is the case with student loans, what shows up on the Web site in the Policy Directives is not a clear indication of how things work in reality. The Ontario Web site indicates that student loans are not considered as income or as assets—with no further clarification. To get clarification, you must have the legislation reviewed by a knowledgeable specialist. Do not rely upon policy directives. Each of the items mentioned is further explained within the legislation; but that legislation, as already noted, is constantly changing.

Integration of other payments

Social assistance payments are generally (in all provinces other than Quebec) *the payors of last resort.* This means that the provincial programs top up any other income streams to reach the minimum level. Therefore, CPP disability benefits, workers' compensation payments, or any other forms of income will be deducted dollar for dollar from provincial social assistance payments. So a person with a disability who has earned the maximum contributory earnings for CPP benefits may well have a CPP disability pension that exceeds the maximum provincial benefit. Combined with workers' compensation, if it was a workplace injury, this means that many people will not receive provincial social assistance payments.

Maximum benefits

The maximum benefit in Ontario, which has not changed since 1998, is made up of several components as follows:

Basic Needs Allowance covers food, clothing, transportation, and all other expenses.

- Single person $516 per month
- Couple $765 per month
- Couple both disabled $1032 per month
- An amount that varies from $110 to $174 per month per child, depending upon the age of the child and the number of children

Shelter Allowance covers rent.

- Single person $414 per month
- Couple $652 per month
- Four people in family $768 per month

Utilities cover the *verifiable actual costs* of natural gas, hydro and water.

There are various other benefits that may be paid on an *as needed* or infrequent basis, such as winter clothing allowances for children and special diets where appropriate.

If the person with a disability is lucky enough to live in a subsidized housing unit, the shelter allowance will be reduced to reflect the actual amount being paid. For example, if the rent subsidy received is $300 per month and the actual rent is $600 per month, the amount of shelter allowance paid will be $300 and not $414 (which is the maximum amount of shelter allowance for a single person). In other words, the maximum amount of the shelter allowance payable will be lower if the actual cost to the person is less than $414.

In the major metropolitan areas, finding a room in a rooming house for $414 per month is difficult. And if the person with the disability uses a wheelchair, that option does not work, since there are unlikely to be wheelchair accessible rooming houses. (Housing issues are covered in more detail in Chapter 14, "Housing Issues for People with Disabilities".)

Other issues

Cohabitation

Common-law spouses of the opposite sex have always been considered to be part of a family unit in Ontario if a financial dependency can be shown.

Same-sex couples are now in the same situation. This could potentially cause problems for people sharing accommodation who are not couples.

At least in Ontario, caseworkers are not allowed to ask about sexual relationships. Only if there appears to be financial interdependence are they allowed to ask about social and family factors, but not sexual relationships. It is therefore important to keep finances as separate as possible if you find yourself sharing accommodation. Have one person pay rent to the other, or split the rent equally. Also split the utilities, phone, cable, etc., equally. Also, separate bank accounts so that one person has no access to the other person's accounts.

Health Benefits

ODSP recipients, and their dependents (known as members of the benefit unit), are automatically eligible for extended health benefits paid by the province. They receive fully paid coverage under this program for drugs, eyeglasses up to a certain amount (not contact lenses), hearing aids and some dental benefits.

Some points to consider:

- ODSP recipients are issued a card for their health benefits that must be presented to receive covered benefits.
- ODSP benefits continue even if you have other income in any given month, provided that you still qualify for a small amount of OSDP benefits, say, $5 per month. So people with disabilities should apply for ODSP benefits even if they are eligible for a very small benefit each month because of the drug benefit. Most people with disabilities require ongoing medication. Although not all drugs needed are covered under the drug formulary of the province, most are. Of course, the applicant must meet income and asset limit tests in order to qualify for ODSP.

Example: Joe has a disability that prevents him from working. He receives CPP benefits totalling $925 per month. His total ODSP entitlement (for housing and personal needs) as a single person is $930 per month. His medication costs $200 per month. By applying for OSDP, his income goes up by only $5 per month, but his expenses for medication will drop by $200 per month. Therefore, the value of the ODSP is $205 per month.

- ODSP also pays for the uncovered portion for assistive devices (See Chapter 15, "Attendant Care and Equipment Funding"), which is typically 25% of the cost, as well as the assessment fee. Other provinces without assistive devices programs usually pay the full cost for people receiving social assistance benefits.
- Some provinces administer disability support programs centrally, through provincial offices.

Others have moved these programs, and other social services, to municipalities.

- For people who have been denied benefits, there are appeal processes in place. However, the process is a minefield of difficulty. The best resource for appeals is a qualified lawyer or a local legal aid clinic.
- Provincial disability income support programs are integrated with other payors (such as CPP/QPP). This puts the provincial programs in the position of last payor (except in Quebec). Since CPP disability payments are indexed to inflation, these payments increase each January. At the same time, ODSP reduces payments by exactly the same amount. Over time, since there have been no increases in ODSP payments since the end of 1997, people with disabilities in Ontario could end up with no further ODSP coverage and could lose their drug/medication benefits as well. With inflation averaging 3% per year, and considering federal benefit indexation, there has been an effective 25% decline in ODSP income since 1997.

Example: Peter has a brain injury and epilepsy. In 1998 he received ODSP of $113 per month with the balance of his income coming from CPP disability payments. In 2003, his ODSP income is $58 per month. The maximum amount he is allowed for medication leaves him with 5 days per year with no drugs—a serious problem for a person with epilepsy. Without an increase in ODSP soon, he will lose ODSP and probably his drug coverage, too.

Employment support programs

Most provinces allow people with disabilities to work part-time and still retain benefits. But the amount that can be earned is quite low. An informal survey of people who work with people with disabilities who are receiving provincial benefits showed a disturbing trend. These professionals said that there is a significant disincentive for people with disabilities to work, since those with high drug costs may lose their health benefits, even if they have relatively low earnings.

Speaking from Experience...
Vocational rehabilitation—a case study

Bob's story

The old system of vocational rehabilitation was quite wonderful, although it was not without problems. But now, when you talk about ODSP and employment support, which is supposed to have taken its place, there is no incentive that I can see for someone with a disability to go back to school to get post-secondary education and eventually find employment.

Bear in mind that a lot of people with spinal cord injuries are young males who have not completed post-secondary education, or even started it. The person with a disability is up against so much already, just by virtue of the disability, that to set up more barriers and make it so difficult for them to access funds to enable them to go to a post-secondary institution with a vocational focus is overwhelming. Without the old system that was in place for me— let me put it this way—I wouldn't be sitting in this office talking to you today, if it weren't for them [the old systems]. And I counsel people through the peer support program and encourage them to go back to school, get new skills, look for work—but in my heart of hearts, I know how incredibly difficult the system is, and the lack of support that is in it.

ODSP does not contribute much to post-secondary education, which means disabled people have to take out student loans. And, of course, it is much more difficult for a person with a disability to find a well-paid job afterwards, and therefore, much more difficult to repay student loans.

Municipal programs

Funding for equipment, such as bath boards, shower chairs, bladder and bowel supplies (incontinence supplies), which are not covered by the provincial Assistive Devices program may, in some cases, be funded by local municipalities in Ontario.

Although ODSP is the same across Ontario, larger municipalities, such as Toronto, have a bigger property tax base and are more prepared and willing to fund such items. This is one reason why people with disabilities gravitate towards large urban centres. The social services departments in these large centres administer such programs. People who are on ODSP or on an Ontario Works program apply for special needs items through the social services department of the municipality.

SOURCES OF INFORMATION

Ontario government benefits — ODSP www.gov.on.ca/CSS/page/brochure/odsips.html

Provincial Government Web sites are listed in the Resources Section at the back of this book.

CHAPTER 9

WORKERS' COMPENSATION

WHAT IS WORKERS' COMPENSATION?

The provincially regulated workers' compensation programs cover on-the-job employee injuries and occupational diseases. These are *no-fault* compensation programs: if an employee is eligible to receive workers' compensation, then the employee *cannot* sue the employer. (If a motor vehicle is involved in the claim, then the employee may be able to sue another party.) Since these programs are not social assistance programs, benefits can be more generous than under provincial social assistance plans.

Workers' compensation plans are administered under provincial legislation that has created specialized boards to oversee the programs. The boards are usually separate from government departments and operate independently under enabling legislation. Every province has different rules and regulations. In the years before workers' compensation plans were introduced, many workers who were injured on the job received no compensation at all for their injuries.

Who Is Covered By Workers' Compensation?

Examples of occupations covered under workers' compensation are those in construction, mining, blasting, oil and gas, diving, fishing or other marine occupations, forestry, wood products and other manufacturing, agriculture, aircraft operations, laboratories, firefighting, occupational first aid and evacuation and rescue. (This summary is extrapolated from the British Columbia Workers' Compensation Board [WCB] Act Excerpts.) But not only employees who are involved in physical work or who are at risk for workplace-related injury and illness, but also most provincial government employees and related services employees are covered by workers' compensation. That is, many "white collar" workers are covered as well. There are some workplaces that are exempt from workers' compensation programs. There are differences from province to province. Most businesses in Ontario that employ workers (including family members and sub-contractors) must register with the Workplace Safety and Insurance Board (WSIB).

A sole proprietor, partner, or executive officer, is not automatically covered under the WSIB insurance plan.

Federal workers are covered under a separate federal government program.

Workers' compensation does *not* cover:

- Workers who are self-employed (though they may purchase optional insurance)
- Those who are working for an employer whose workplace is not covered under worker's compensation
- Those who injure themselves on their own time

In Ontario, there are a few industries that do not have to register, although they may do so if they wish. These include the following:

- Banks, trusts and insurance companies
- Private health care practices (such as those of doctors and chiropractors)
- Trade unions
- Private day care centres
- Travel agencies
- Clubs (such as health clubs)
- Photographers
- Barbers, hair salons, and shoe-shine stands
- Taxidermists
- Funeral directing and embalming

To be eligible to receive benefits, claimants must have suffered an injury, disease, or impairment directly related to their work.

What Benefits Are Available To Workers Under The Plan?

There are many types of claims that can be brought under workers' compensation plans. Typical benefits include the following:

- Loss of earnings
- Loss of retirement income
- Health care benefits
- Survivor benefits
- Benefits for seriously injured workers
- Death benefits

The most important thing to do is to file a report and claim as soon as possible after the disabling event. The benefits payable depend upon the nature of the claim and the coverage provided through each provincial workers' compensation plan. As such, the services and benefits are too complex to detail in this chapter. Fortunately, each province has a Web site with detailed information. (See the listing of provincial offices and Web sites for workers' compensation at the end of this chapter.)

How are Workers' Compensation Plans Funded and Managed?

Employers fund the workers' compensation plans through premiums based on a number of factors, including the following:

- A general or base rate for all workplaces
- The number of workers in the workplace whose work qualifies them to be covered under the plan
- The type of work performed at the workplace
- Estimates of the extent of possible claims during a year (Some industries have higher rates of risk, and therefore, premiums are higher.)

- The number of claims made from a particular company in the past.

Workers' Compensation plans are administered by Boards empowered under provincial legislation. Each province has such legislation, and the name of the Board differs from province to province.

Seriously Injured Workers

Since space does not permit a province-by-province or category-by-category description of workers' compensation benefits, this section gives an overview of possible benefits and allowances for seriously injured workers in Ontario. Other provinces have similar provisions, but each province has different levels of coverage and conditions for eligibility.

Seriously injured workers are defined in Ontario as workers in the following circumstances:

- Hemiplegia, paraplegia, quadriplegia, or paraparesis
- Major amputations (defined as indicating bodily impairment of more than 60%, which would generally result from amputation of more than a single limb)
- Blindness
- Burns (defined as second or third degree burns involving both hands and feet, or the face, head or neck area; or burns that required the worker to be transferred to a major burn unit)
- Brain injuries that require major cognitive interventions, prevent the worker from living independently, or prevent the worker from handling their own affairs
- Serious crushing injuries to chest, abdomen, or pelvis such as those requiring transfer to a major trauma hospital

Ontario puts out a WSIB publication called "Your Guide to Independent Living" (publication 2264A 07/01), in which the seriously injured employee is specifically requested not to share it with other workers since it applies *only* to those workers who are seriously disabled.

In Ontario, the *Serious Injury Adjudicator* must approve a *Serious Injury Claim*. Seriously injured workers in Ontario may be assigned an *Independent Living Consultant*, an *Advanced Practice Nurse Case Manager*, and a *Special Needs Controller*. Each of these people is responsible for overseeing different areas of benefits.

Possible benefits for injured workers (especially seriously injured workers)

In Ontario, the benefit scheme changed January 1, 1998. In brief, WSIB (and most workers' compensation boards) pay the following types of benefits, which are indexed to inflation. The following benefits are available to all injured workers who meet the entitlement criteria.

- *Loss of earnings and impairment benefits.* This benefit is based on a percentage of previous take-home pay. It is a non-taxable benefit because the employer pays the premium. There is a maximum payment based on an annual wage ceiling, above which benefits paid are capped. The benefits paid can depend upon the date of the start of injury or impairment. Many people covered under workers' compensation are also covered by group disability policies. In such cases, there is likely a clause in the group policy that deducts workers' compensation payments from group disability payouts on a dollar-for-dollar basis.

- *Loss of retirement income benefits.* To ensure that workers who are disabled do not have low incomes in their retirement years, this benefit, in effect, ensures that a percentage of the loss of earnings amount is invested and then used to fund a retirement income benefit. (In Ontario, for example, after 12 months of disability under workers' compensation, 5% of the loss of earnings amount is automatically contributed to the Loss of Retirement Income Benefits account on behalf of the worker.) Workers can contribute an additional 5% of their loss of earnings benefit. Prior to 1998, workers' compensation in Ontario set aside the full 10%.

- *Non-economic loss benefit.* This benefit may be awarded if the injury or illness is severe enough to cause permanent impairment. The amount of the benefit is based on the seriousness of the impairment and the age of the claimant, and is to compensate for physical, psychological, and functional loss caused by the impairment once no further improvement is expected. Calculations are complex. The payment may be awarded as a lump sum or as a monthly annuity for the remainder of the claimant's life.
- *Survivor benefits.* This benefit is awarded in cases where an injured worker, who is 100% disabled, dies.
- *Health care benefits.* These benefits cover costs such as prescription drugs, medical devices, transportation costs associated with medical treatment, and are available to all workers depending upon their circumstances.

If the serious injury occurred in Ontario before 1998, benefits are subject to an established indexation formula.

Additional benefits for seriously injured workers in Ontario

Although the benefits described below are most frequently provided to the most seriously injured workers, those with less serious injuries may qualify for some of these benefits in some situations.

- *Attendant's allowance.* If you need assistance with the activities of daily living (such as washing, dressing, feeding yourself), you may hire an attendant to provide assistance. WSIB will pay a monthly allowance depending on your assessed needs. If you need care more than 24 hours per week, you will be considered to be an employer of the attendant. It is similar to self-funded attendant care. (See Chapter 15, "Attendant Care Services and Equipment Funding.") Friends or family may help with hiring and directing care.
- *Clothing allowance.* This benefit covers wear and tear on clothing caused by the need to use a wheelchair or certain prosthetic devices, braces, and other assistive devices. Payment depends on how many hours per week the device is needed.
- *Independent living allowance.* This benefit covers home maintenance costs, yard maintenance and snow shovelling, recreational and group therapy programs, independent living devices including items to assist with communication such as telephones and computers, specialty hospital beds, easy-lift chairs, motorized scooters, and other devices. In most cases, to be eligible for this benefit, you must be 100% permanently disabled.
- *Guide and support dog allowance.* This allowance, worth up to $820 per year for 2002 is available to workers who are profoundly deaf, visually impaired, or who have significant mobility needs as a result of their workplace injury.
- *Travel and escort payments.* These payments pay transportation for attending WSIB meetings and appointments. Payments can be for parking, travelling, hotel bills, and meals, if approved by WSIB.
- *Quality of life, sports and hobby activities benefit.* This benefit covers the purchase of special devices to assist in pursuit of various interests, including elevator installation to access another floor of the

house to participate in family activities and the purchase of special devices to pursue hobbies

Tax and Other Implications of Workers' Compensation Payments

Although workers' compensation benefits are non-taxable, they are part of your net income and must be reported on your tax return. They will potentially affect any refundable tax credits (such as GST tax credit, child tax benefit, and provincial tax benefits), as well as lowering the amount you can claim for medical expenses. A T5007 will be issued each year for workers compensation benefits paid during the year. Other payments, such as interest, non-economic loss awards, medical expenses, survivor's lump-sum payments and burial expenses are not included in income and are not taxable.

Some people with disabilities collect provincial social assistance benefits or disability insurance benefits while they are waiting for the workers' compensation board to evaluate their claim. These amounts are treated as advances. The workers' compensation board reimburses those agencies once the claim is paid.

Benefits are available to a maximum of age 65, at which time, the retirement income benefit will start, if applicable.

Appeals

There is an appeal process in the event that the claimant does not agree with a decision by the WSIB (or other provincial workers' compensation board). These appeal routes will vary by province. There are also specialty legal clinics in several provinces as well as the regular legal aid clinics. The provincial Web sites have a lot of information and descriptions of the appeals process. Check with your local legal aid clinic or contact your provincial Law Society for the telephone number of the legal aid clinic nearest you.

Example of a serious injury claim and award in Ontario:

Fred suffered a fall at work in Ontario and as a result has quadriplegia. Since he is a seriously injured worker, he receives the following benefits from WSIB:

- A lifetime monthly benefit
- Contribution to the retirement income fund
- Payment for an attendant
- Payment for the cost of a modified, wheelchair accessible van
- Payment for the cost of an electric wheelchair and a manual wheelchair for use in the home
- Payment for all aids and supplies required
- Money to build a two-storey addition with an elevator to enable him to continue living in his own home

What Happens If a Recipient Moves Out of Province or Out of Canada?

If an injured worker voluntarily moves to another province or relocates outside of Canada, there may be negative repercussions. This particularly applies to relocation outside of Canada. For example, according to the Saskatchewan Workers' Compensation Board Web site:

- Payments will no longer be made by electronic funds transfer.
- Benefits and expenses will be paid only in Canadian funds.
- Medical expenses will be paid at Saskatchewan provincial health plan rates.
- A re-evaluation of your ability to earn a living is required at the time of the move and annually thereafter (if receiving the benefits for loss of earnings based on an estimation of your earnings capacity).
- Any needed medical or vocational rehabilitation plan must be established before relocating.

- Suspension or termination of benefits can occur if, as a result of relocating, active medical treatment or rehabilitation plans are disrupted.
- After you relocate, you're responsible for obtaining and paying for any translation of medical and other reports that are required by the Workers' Compensation Board.
- Travel expenses will be calculated and paid for as if you had continued to live in Saskatchewan.
- Yearly verification of your residency and competency will be required.

In short, be very careful about relocating and obtain approval first. When relocating to another province, there will be a waiting period before provincial benefits such as health care start. (See Chapter 16, "Miscellany: After Care, Home Care, Caregiving Issues".)

According to statistics provided by the Labour Branch of Human Resources Development Canada, the number of people on workers' compensation benefits across Canada has steadily declined since 1989, when there were a total of 615,929. By 1997, which is the last year for which numbers are available as preliminary figures, this had declined to 399,542. This is the lowest number for more than 20 years. Of course, whether this is related to a tightening of claims criteria or an improvement in workplace safety is unknown.

In Quebec, there is a higher number of workers' compensation claims per year than Ontario, but only about one third the number of QPP disability claims. This is probably because the QPP plan is administered differently and workers with disabilities are channelled into the workers' compensation program.

Commentary

Although compensation for workplace injuries and disabilities has been improved thanks to workers' compensation plans, there are still some troubling aspects to the coverage. Since employers must pay for the coverage, they are anxious to keep their premiums low. They therefore wish to have as few employees on claim for as short a period as possible. The employer is supposed to offer a "suitable" job to a worker who is recovering from injury or illness. The advice of the worker's medical doctor is supposed to be considered. Anecdotal reports suggest, however, that after a disability some injured employees return to jobs that have not been modified to help the injured worker build up to their pre-injury level of strength or skill: they are the same jobs that caused the injuries in the first place. Often, requested intervention by union representatives does not help the worker, either.

In some provinces, workers' compensation program are shifting their emphasis to *prevention* rather than *treatment*. While laudable, the fact still remains that workers do get injured on the job despite all the training on job safety.

As with any type of "insurance," once a claim is made, the individual is in an adversarial relationship with the insuring body. Mediation is a feature of the system in all provinces. Although appeals of decisions can be made, once the final appeal panel decides, there is no further avenue open to the injured worker. Note that there can be several levels of appeals depending upon provincial legislation. Since these are no-fault insurance programs, the employee cannot sue the employer for further damages. Workers' compensation programs are *non-recourse* programs: once the highest level of appeal body has ruled on the claim, the claimant can take no further action.

APPENDIX A:

Examples of Worker Hazards Covered under Workers' Compensation Plans: (Extrapolated from the British Columbia WCB Act Excerpts and Summaries)

- Chemical and biological substances
- Substance specific requirements
- Noise, vibration, radiation and temperature
- Personal protective clothing and equipment
- Confined spaces
- Fall protection
- Tools, machinery and equipment
- Ladders, scaffolds and temporary work platforms
- Cranes and hoists
- Rigging
- Mobile equipment
- Transportation of workers
- Traffic control
- Electrical safety

SOURCES OF INFORMATION

How to contact Provincial Workers' Compensation Boards

WORKERS' COMPENSATION
BOARD OF ALBERTA
P.O. Box 2415
9912-107 Street
Edmonton AB T5J 2S5
Tel: 780-498-4000
Fax: 780-498-7875
http: www.wcb.ab.ca

WORKERS' COMPENSATION
BOARD OF BRITISH
COLUMBIA
P.O. Box 5350
Vancouver BC V6B 5L5
Tel: 604-273-2266
Fax: 604-276-3151
http: www.worksafebc.com

WORKERS' COMPENSATION
BOARD OF MANITOBA
333 Broadway
Winnipeg MB R3C 4W3
Tel: 204-954-4321
Fax: 204-954-4968
http: www.wcb.mb.ca

WORKPLACE HEALTH,
SAFETY AND COMPENSATION
COMMISSION
1 Portland Street
P.O. Box 160
Saint John NB E2L 3X9
Tel: 506-632-2200
Fax: 506-632-4999
http: www.whscc.nb.ca

WORKPLACE HEALTH SAFETY
AND COMPENSATION
COMMISSION
146-148 Forest Road
P.O. Box 9000, Station B
St. John's NF A1A 3B8
Tel: 709-778-1000
Fax: 709-738-1714
http: www.whscc.nf.ca

WORKERS' COMPENSATION
BOARD OF THE NORTHWEST
TERRITORIES AND NUNAVUT
P.O. Box 8888
Yellowknife NT X1A 2R3
Tel: 867-920-3888
Fax: 867-873-4596
http: www.wcb.nt.ca

WORKERS' COMPENSATION
BOARD OF NOVA SCOTIA
5668 South Street
P.O. Box 1150
Halifax NS B3J 2Y2
Tel: 902-491-8999
Fax: 902-491-8002
http: www.wcb.ns.ca

WORKPLACE SAFETY AND
INSURANCE BOARD (Ontario)
200 Front Street West
Toronto ON M5V 3J1
Tel: 416-344-1000
Fax: 416-344-3999
http: www.wsib.on.ca

WORKERS' COMPENSATION
BOARD OF PRINCE EDWARD
ISLAND
14 Weymouth Street
Charlottetown PEI C1A 4Y1
Tel: 902-368-5680
Fax: 902-368-5705
http: www.wcb.pe.ca

COMMISSION DE LA SANTÉ
ET DE LA SÉCURITÉ DU
TRAVAIL
1199, rue de Bleury
C.P. 6056,
Succursale «Centre-Ville»
Montréal QC H3C 4E1
Tel: 514-906-3780
Fax: 514-906-3781
http: www.csst.qc.ca

WORKERS' COMPENSATION
BOARD OF SASKATCHEWAN
200, 1881 Scarth Street
Regina SK S4P 4L1
Tel: 306-787-4370
Fax: 306-787-0213
http: www.wcbsask.com

YUKON WORKERS'
COMPENSATION HEALTH &
SAFETY BOARD
401 Strickland Street
Whitehorse YK Y1A 5N8
Tel: 867-667-5645
Fax: 867-393-6279
http: www.wcb.yk.ca

ASSOCIATION OF WORKERS'
COMPENSATION BOARDS
(A national organization):
www.awcbc.org

CHAPTER 10

DISABILITY AND THE SELF-EMPLOYED SMALL BUSINESS PERSON

Note that the "ground rules" for disability insurance are covered in Chapter 4, "Disability Insurance." This chapter discusses particular concerns for the self-employed small business person.

In this chapter, the focus is on individuals who are currently self-employed or are small business owners, who are concerned with preventive action in case disability does occur.

UNINCORPORATED SOLE PROPRIETORSHIP

An unincorporated sole proprietorship is the simplest form of business ownership. It means that the business is an extension of the person as an individual for tax and legal purposes. The income and expenses of the business are reported in a special section of the personal income tax return. Standard personal tax advantages are available to the individual business owner.

Unless a business has operations that may give rise to legal liability issues, there is little value, in terms of tax benefits, to incorporating until the profit (income after business expenses) from the business is at least $100,000 per year. The extent of an individual's liability, the type of business, and the assets exposed to ongoing liability issues should also be part of the decision of whether or not to incorporate—not just tax considerations.

The amount of disability insurance that the sole proprietor can purchase is based on the net income from the business. This is normally averaged over a 3-year period. The amount of coverage is normally two thirds of net income averaged over the previous 3 years as reported on tax returns. Some adjustments may be made to this average. For example, owners who use a personally owned vehicle for business and who write off a portion of those costs on their tax returns may be able to add those amounts back in calculating net income for disability insurance purposes. This adjustment can also apply to home office expenses and medical insurance premiums paid through the business. But most insurance companies work with the bottom line as verified by the Notice of Assessment from Canada Customs and Revenue Agency (CCRA), formerly Revenue Canada.

The amount of benefit received at the time of a claim will be tax-free since the individual pays the premiums as a sole proprietor. This means that the amount of income coverage required (benefit amount) can be kept to a reasonable level, and therefore the insurance premium can be kept at reasonable cost.

Difficulties in Obtaining Disability Insurance for the Self-employed

- It can sometimes take several years (6 years is not uncommon) after a business has been started before any substantial net income appears on the tax return.
- Those small business owners who are extra zealous in taking tax deductions can reduce their net income to a point where they minimize the amount of coverage to which they will be entitled— to their disadvantage.
- If the self-employed person has left a position with a large private or public employer which offered substantial benefits, they will have additional costs in replacing those benefits. Sometimes, business owners do not take into account the cost of disability insurance, life insurance, and extended health benefits in estimating the cost structure of their own small business.

- In some cases, there is provision for the total amount of insurance to be paid up to a maximum of 85% of pre-disability earnings starting on a graduated scale. Certain professionals, such as lawyers, doctors and dentists, who are working in group practices, often set up additional (often called *top hat*) coverage that can increase the amount of benefits to $10,000 per month.

Tips for Obtaining Disability Insurance for the Self-employed Person

If you are employed, have disability coverage through your employer, and are thinking of starting your own business, or are thinking of becoming self-employed at some point in the future, consider taking out an individual policy *in addition* to the group coverage. This provides a basic level of protection regardless of your employment. Review Chapter 4, "Disability Insurance."

- As a self-employed person, consider obtaining disability insurance through a group plan, such as an alumni association, professional organization, or a local Board of Trade or Chamber of Commerce. This will allow you to benefit from the group rate and ensure that you have some protection.
- If you are planning to become self-employed soon, or are concerned that you may lose your job in the future, purchase your own private disability insurance *now*. In this way, you will be prepared. The amount of coverage will be based on your income level now, not in the future. Insurance companies co-ordinate benefits so that you do not receive more than 75% to 80% of your pre-disability income, if you have a claim, regardless of which plans you have at work or which you purchase privately.
- If you are taking out a loan, especially if you are unsure of your employment prospects for the duration of the loan, consider taking out disability

insurance on that loan, if you are eligible. Since it is about three to four times more likely that you could become disabled rather than die during the term of the loan, such coverage makes sense.

- If you can purchase your own individual disability insurance, be sure that you understand the basics of disability insurance policies as covered in Chapter 4, "Disability Insurance." The important points to remember include:
  — The definition of occupation
  — Residual income versus partial income benefits
  — Length of coverage
  — Waiver of premium
  — Return of premium
  — Cost of living allowance

At a minimum, purchase 60 months of *regular occupation or own occupation by virtue of training, education and experience coverage.*

INCORPORATED BUSINESSES

An advantage to an incorporated business is that income can be deferred from one year to the next. This is done by controlling the amount of salary or dividends paid to the company's owners each year. Since the corporation is a separate legal entity, there is some (but not total) protection from certain legal actions taken against the firm's owners and shareholders.

Disability insurance on corporate owners or directors can be purchased personally or by the corporation.

If you purchase the disability insurance personally, then you receive tax-free benefits if you have a disability claim. The amount of coverage that you can purchase depends upon the amount of your salary or income, generally averaged over several years. If you make a claim, the insurance company will ask for income verification over a 5-year period or on a month-to-month basis for the previous 12 months.

If you buy the disability insurance through the corporation on behalf of the individual, then the benefits, when received, are taxable. This tax liability means that a higher amount of coverage must be purchased.

With taxable disability benefits, the amount received is considered to be earned income for RRSP purposes. Therefore, RRSP contributions can be made based on this income. This assumes that you will have income from other assets and will not need the maximum after-tax amount of the disability benefit just to meet living expenses. For example, if you have other sources of taxable income, such as that from investments or a rental property, you could possibly cover both living expenses and the cost of making RRSP contributions. Since disability insurance payments stop at age 65, there is an advantage to building up an RRSP to add to long term retirement income after age 65.

If the corporation owns the disability policy, and if the business owner sells the corporation, the individual may not have disability coverage after the sale. Provisions should therefore be incorporated into the Buy–Sell Agreement and/or into the Shareholders Agreement to ensure protection and stipulate what the individual would receive. When there is more than one owner of the corporation, a solution is for the owners of the business to have disability coverage for themselves and key employees purchased by the corporation, with other policies that the individuals own and pay for personally. The privately owned policies continue in force separate from the corporation's policies. Assuming that the group (corporate) policy continues for 2 years, with *own occupation* coverage, the individual policies would be taken out with waiting periods of 24 months (2 years) or with lower benefits, and lower costs, over that time period. The individually owned policies would then increase benefits beginning after 24 months when the group plan's own occupation coverage ends.

What to Consider When Buying Disability Insurance as a Sole Proprietor or Incorporated Business Owner

- Can the business survive without you? If yes, for how long?
- Do you have cash reserves or an emergency fund in the business that can keep it afloat for a period of time? Would the reserves last at least 6 months? This means paying all expenses including a draw or income to yourself.
- Do you have receivables in your business that will also keep the business afloat for a period of time? For how long?
- Do you have a succession plan in place to cover these eventualities?
  — If you should die
  — If your partner should die
  — If you or your partner should suffer a disability
  — If you or your partner should want to retire early
  — If you operate your business with your spouse, would he or she want to continue to run the business without you? Would he or she be able to do so?
  — Will the business have to be sold in the event of a disability —and would there be a buyer for it? Would it have any value without you? Does your Power of Attorney for Property have a specific clause to address how the business should be handled?
  — Are there any assets in the business that could be sold, such as major equipment, vehicles, a building, etc.?
  — Do you have Office Overhead Insurance? (See next section)

Receiving Disability Income at Claims Time

The general principles of claims payout discussed in Chapter 4, "Disability Insurance" apply here. But there are special features that can apply to self-employed business persons' policies. The most important feature is that for *residual income benefits*. This is a rider on the policy and there is an additional cost.

After returning to work, net business income may be significantly reduced because:

- the owner has ongoing residual effects from the disability;
- income has been lost during the period of the disability; and/or
- income may fluctuate from month to month, so that some months the business owner may not be eligible for benefits, but in other months full or partial benefits may be payable.

The advantage to *Residual income benefits* is that, as your income fluctuates when you return to work, the *residual income rider* will either pay out benefits (up to the policy maximum) or will reduce the dollar value of the benefits received if your monthly income exceeds the maximum that is based on your earnings before the disability.

Residual income benefits for ongoing partial disability can be covered until age 65 or to the end of the term of the policy, with monthly adjustments according to how much net business income loss there has been in that month.

How are Residual Income Benefits Calculated?

Your pre-disability earnings are based on your income after you have paid your business expenses. In most cases, *residual income benefits* equal to the full amount of insurance coverage will continue to be paid as long as net income after expenses is less than 20% of pre-disability earnings. This is sometimes phrased as an income loss of at least 80% of pre-disability earnings. Once the person's net income is at 80% of pre-disability earnings, no benefits will be payable for that month. In between the 20% and 80%, income from the disability insurance will be based on the percentage loss of income.

For example, if a self-employed person's pre-disability net income (gross income less business expenses) was $4,000 per month and they have coverage for $2,000 per month, then net business earnings of $1,000 per month (25% of the pre-disability income) during this residual period would reduce the disability payment by 25% or $500 per month.

If you take a *cost of living adjustment* (COLA) as part of the policy, not only will the maximum benefit payable be increased each year on the anniversary date, but also the pre-disability earnings calculation will be increased by the same percentage. However, as with all policies, there are variations—not just between insurance companies, but also between different disability insurance plans within the same company. It is important to check the actual wording in your own policy and to understand all the benefits to which you are entitled and to ensure that you receive them.

Recordkeeping for residual income benefit payout

Of course, this benefit requires that you keep accurate records of income and expenses on a monthly basis. Many people find this very onerous. These accounts must be submitted to the insurance company monthly before your benefit for that month will be payable the next month.

The monthly report includes this information:

- Income from earnings, employment, business or corporate profit, dividends and loans, or any other earned income.
- All expenses, including amortization or depreciation, payroll taxes, home office expenses,

(if eligible) and any other expenses you would normally deduct in the course of operating your business.

- Copies of all expenses such as telephone bills, office supplies, car expenses, and rent.

If the person with the disability did the bookkeeping before the disability, but can no longer do so, then someone has to be hired to do this on a monthly basis. This is often a cause of some frustration for the person with a disability—especially if they are making so little that it is a financial hardship to hire a bookkeeper to help them.

Most insurance companies will require copies of the previous 5 years' tax returns (including the Notice of Assessment for each year) or a month-by-month breakdown and earnings for the 12 months immediately before the disabling event, in order to calculate monthly pre-disability income.

Each year, a copy of the current year's tax return will be required by the insurance company to verify income reported.

BUSINESS OVERHEAD INSURANCE

Business overhead insurance provides specific insurance that is designed to cover the *overhead costs* of a business in the event of the owner's or key person's disability. It is valuable in that the business then has income flowing into it to maintain the office premises and related office expenses. In addition, the inflow of funds provides a period of adjustment until you know the extent of the disability and can arrange for the ongoing management of the business.

Business overhead insurance covers such items as:
- Rent or office lease costs
- Telephone service
- Equipment rental or leases

- Key personnel payroll costs (often covered by *key person insurance* as a rider or separate policy)
- Other office expenses according to the policy document, which might include: professional dues, accounting services, liability insurance, certain taxes, office supplies, some office expenses, equipment depreciation, etc.

Usually, the amount covered is about 80% of expenses, which is paid out for no more than 18 to 36 months. Ideally, you would purchase *business overhead insurance* to cover the length of time remaining on a commercial office lease.

There are some restrictions on obtaining *business overhead insurance*:

- If your spouse or other family member is employed by your firm and is in effect performing administrative or back-up services, the chances are that the overhead insurance would not cover that person's salary.
- For home-based businesses, it is more difficult to obtain business overhead insurance, although the amount of overhead may be lower than that for commercial office space.

Costs of Business Overhead Insurance

The costs for *business overhead insurance* depend on the elements in the package selected, and on the number, age and occupations (non-sales staff) of the employees covered. For example, an employer with two employees, (age 45 and under), could buy modest coverage for under $400 per month. This would include the following:

- $25,000 of life insurance and accidental death and dismemberment
- A weekly indemnity from the 15th day of disability up to 15 weeks

Long term disability insurance from the 121st day of disability to age 65 for $2,250 per month
- Critical illness coverage of $25,000 reducing to $12,000 at age 55
- Business overhead insurance of $1,000 per month of benefit

Not covered in this example are dependent life insurance, extended health coverage, or dental coverage. This coverage is a group package covering several employees—not individual business overhead insurance.

As with all types of disability insurance, it is important to contact an insurance professional who can advise you on the best plan for your own situation.

KEY PERSON INSURANCE

Insurance coverage for a particular individual in a business for disability or death is often referred to as *key person insurance*. The insurance policy can be owned by the individual who is insured, by the business for which the insured person works, or by a partner or partners with whom the individual works in the firm.

The coverage in a partnership, in particular, can be "criss-cross" coverage. That is, one partner owns the policy on the life of the other partner and vice versa. In the event of disability or death, the policy on the person with a disability or deceased partner pays out funds to the owner of the policy. In the event of disability, the policy pays out money to the firm so that another individual can be hired to temporarily take over the job function of the person who has been disabled.

PRIVATE HEALTH SERVICE PLANS (Health and Welfare Trusts)

Private health service plans, available to both unincorporated and incorporated businesses, fall under

Section 248 (1) of the Income Tax Act, which allows for Health and Welfare Trusts. It is a means of self-insuring medical and dental expenses and the coverage may be much broader than what is available in most off-the-shelf plans. This type of plan is set up under a trust agreement that outlines the various conditions of the plan.

The Private Health Service Plan (PHSP) covers group supplementary or extended health benefits. Instead of buying such group coverage off-the-shelf from an insurance company, the business owners set up their own plan for coverage through an accredited insurance broker or trustee. Coverage under the PHSP is broader than what is offered through off-the-shelf supplementary or extended health plans.

The PHSP is not for life insurance or disability coverage.

The PHSP covers both management and employees for such services as dental care, vision care, prescriptions, physiotherapy, laboratory tests, contraceptives, pre and post-natal care, gynecology, therapy equipment, insulin, and so on. (See the Income Tax Act, Section 118.2 for a complete list.)

The coverage is basically for all medically necessary expenses as ordered by a medical or qualified health care practitioner. Fully 100% of the qualifying expenses or health service costs incurred can be claimed from the plan. There does not have to be a deductible amount on claims under these plans. But employers can limit the claim costs in other ways such as setting up a *health plan voucher account* for each employee, so that there is a dollar value to benefits provided for each employee in a calendar year. The costs of these plans are usually deductible by the business.

Business owners who want to set up PHSPs must be actively engaged alone, or in partnership, in a business from which they derive their primary source of income as income from self-employment. In short, the income from the business must be more than 50% of the person's income. Furthermore, the total income from other sources cannot be greater than $10,000 per year.

In setting up the plan, the employer must provide equal coverage to all full-time employees who are at arm's length from the employer (that is, people who are not related to the employer).

Unincorporated business owners can contribute up to $1,500 per year for each worker and his or her spouse (that's $3,000 per year), and $750 per child. In an unincorporated business, if there are at least an equal number of employees who are not related to the owners to be covered under the plan, then there are no contribution limits and as much funding as needed can be put into the trust to keep it operating.

For incorporated businesses, there is no contribution limit per employee.

These contribution amounts are deductible from the income of the business. There is no taxable benefit to the employee covered under the plan.

Administratively, the funds in the PHSP must be segregated in a trust, separate from the company's other funds.

A concern with the PHSP is excessive use of the plan by employees: this is why some employers give employees a *health plan voucher account* that allows the employee to make claims up to a certain dollar amount per year and based on certain conditions. Pre-funding the PHSP is another option where the employer contributes, for example, $2,000 per employee per year to the PHSP rather than paying on a claims-made basis The costs of setting up such a PHSP can be under $500, with an annual administrative fee in the range of 10% to 15% of claims paid.

As with any plan, expert advice is required. Contact a life insurance agent or broker who specializes in this area.

OTHER THINGS TO CONSIDER

Canada Pension Plan Disability Benefits

In order to receive maximum Canada Pension Plan disability benefits, the individual claimant must have had net business income or salary of about $40,000 per year for 4 out of the last 6 years. (See Chapter 7, "Federal Government Benefits.")

Critical Illness and Long Term Care Policies

Critical illness coverage is an option for a self-employed person who cannot get disability insurance, or who wants to expand coverage beyond what is available in a disability policy. (See Chapter 6, "Critical Illness and Long Term-Care Insurance.")

Supplementary Health Care (Extended Health) Benefits and Other Insurance Options

As outlined in Chapter 5, "Employee Benefit and Individual Plans," supplementary health care benefits may be part of an employer plan, or they may be purchased privately. One-person companies, partnerships, entrepreneurs and small companies can access these plans, too. Often, there are pre-determined packages of benefits available. Life and health insurance brokers also offer custom-designed plans.

Self-employed individuals can deduct all of their premiums for extended health care/supplementary health care coverage from their annual income.

SOURCES OF INFORMATION

Canadian Life and Health Insurance Association (CLHIA): www.clhia.ca Go to the Consumer Assistance Centre button on the site for information on extended health benefit/ supplementary health benefit companies.

Specific extended health benefit/supplemental health benefit and optional insurance companies and distributors have Web sites or can be contacted through a qualified life and health insurance agent. (See also CLHIA above.)

CHAPTER 11

THE INCOME TAX SYSTEM AND PEOPLE WITH DISABILITIES

The Canadian income tax system, as administered by Canada Customs and Revenue Agency (CCRA—formerly Revenue Canada), is based on the idea that all income is taxable—with the exceptions outlined in the Income Tax Act. These exceptions are the basis of how tax laws are applied. It's like a contest: you qualify for certain exceptions if you have met certain basic criteria. You don't qualify or get tax relief if you haven't met the criteria. Of most interest to Canadians with disabilities are *tax deductions* and *tax credits.* Tax deductions are calculated to reduce your net income, the amount on which taxes are calculated. Once the amount of tax you owe has been determined, tax credits are applied to reduce that amount.

The tax system in general strives to recognize and alleviate tax burdens faced by Canadians who are disabled. Not all Canadians with disabilities will qualify for all the possible benefits, but Canadians with severe disabilities and their families will receive most, if not all, the possible credits and deductions that are available to disabled taxpayers.

Most of the provisions in this chapter are federal and apply to all Canadian residents with some variations by province. Residents of Quebec may be entitled to additional credits on their provincial tax returns.

When is Income from a Disability Insurance Plan Taxable?

As discussed in Chapter 4, "Disability Insurance," income from group or individual disability insurance plans is *tax-free* if the employee or individual paid for the premiums on their own. If the employer paid for all or part of the premiums, then disability benefits when received will be *taxable.*

Monies received as the result of a legal settlement (See Chapter 12, "Legal Settlement Options") are not taxable as a lump sum—*but* the income received as a result of investing that lump sum *is* taxable unless it is received as a structured settlement.

The Disability Tax Credit

The disability tax credit, also called the disability amount, is a non-refundable tax credit available to people who meet the following criteria:

- They are blind all, or almost all, of the time even with the use of corrective lenses or medication, and the impairment is *prolonged*
- They have a *severe* and *prolonged* mental or physical impairment that markedly restricts their ability to perform a *basic activity of daily living.*
- They need, and dedicate time specifically for, *life-sustaining therapy* to support a vital function.

The definition of a *prolonged impairment* is one that has lasted, or can reasonably be expected to last, for a continuous period of at least 12 months. Therefore, something that causes a disability that is intermittent is *not* considered to be prolonged.

The *basic activities of daily living* are defined as

- Perceiving
- Thinking and remembering
- Feeding and dressing
- Speaking, hearing
- Eliminating bodily waste
- Walking

The basic activities of daily living *do not include:*

- Working
- Housekeeping
- Recreation or social activities

An activity *may qualify* if all, or most all of the time, the person is unable (or takes an extremely long time) to complete a basic activity of daily living even with therapy and the use of assistive devices and medication.

Life-sustaining therapy does *not* include implanted devices such as pacemakers or special programs of diet, exercise, hygiene or medication.

However, it *does* include clapping therapy to help with breathing and kidney dialysis to filter blood. For 2000 and later years, individuals may qualify if the medical doctor certifies that they need, and must dedicate time specifically for life-sustaining therapy, at least 3 times a week to an average of at least 14 hours a week. Again, the need for this therapy must have lasted, or be expected to last, for a continuous period of at least 12 months.

The amount of the federal disability tax credit is $6,180 in 2002 and is indexed to inflation. If you live in New Brunswick, Manitoba, Yukon, Northwest Territories or Nunavut, the provincial or territorial disability tax credit will be the same amount. In all the other provinces, there is a separate calculation for all non-refundable tax credits, including those for disability, so that the amount of the credit will vary from province to province.

There are two important things to remember about the federal disability amount. Firstly, this is a *non-refundable tax credit*. This means that, if the person making the claim has very little income, there is no benefit from the disability tax credit. However, you may be able to transfer this amount to a spouse, parent or other supporting person who does have taxable income. Secondly, the amount that the disability tax credit is worth is approximately 24% or $1,480 as a credit against tax owing in 2002. It will vary according to the province of residence and the tax bracket of the person making the claim.

Federal disability supplement

If the person with a disability is under 18, there is also a federal disability supplement that applies in all provinces (except in Newfoundland). The amount of this credit for 2002 is up to $3,605. This amount is reduced by any claims for childcare and attendant care that are more than $2,112 for the dependent.

How to claim the disability amount

To claim the disability tax credit, Form T2201 must be completed and submitted with the income tax return for the year when first making a claim. This form may be completed by someone else on behalf of the person with the disability if he or she is unable to do so themselves. Part of the form has to be completed by a certified practitioner who is one of the following:

- A medical doctor, or
- An optometrist for a vision impairment, or
- An audiologist for a hearing impairment, or
- An occupational therapist for a feeding dressing or walking impairment, or
- A speech and language pathologist for a speech impairment

Note: *Just because someone receives a disability pension, this does not mean that they automatically qualify for the disability tax credit.*

CCRA has tightened up considerably on disability tax credit claims in the past few years. Even people who have been using wheelchairs for the past 20 years or who have an ongoing or congenital disability that means that they have always required constant care and attention, are being asked to resubmit disability tax credit forms on a fairly frequent basis.

As an example, people who have had multiple sclerosis for a number of years are receiving renewals for only 2 years on their disability tax credit form. The reason provided by CCRA is that treatments change and that for conditions that were untreatable in the past, there may now be medications or procedures to alleviate the problem. (No doubt many patients would like to know what tax assessors know that they don't!)

There is usually a fee charged by a medical professional for the completion of the form T2201. This cost is the responsibility of the person with a disability, but it can be claimed as a medical expense on the income tax return.

Even when all the eligibility criteria have been met for a disability tax credit, there are still other restrictions that may apply. These will be discussed later in the chapter.

Medical Expenses

Medical expenses are also a non-refundable tax credit, but the credit is not necessarily the same for everybody. The credit is calculated as a percentage of the total amount of medical expenses after deducting 3% of net income (up to a maximum deduction of $1,728 in 2002) from line 236 of the personal income tax return.

For example, if your net income in 2002 was $10,000, and your medical expenses were $2,000, the amount that is eligible for the non-refundable tax credit is $1,700, because $2,000 minus $300 (3% of $10,000) is $1,700.

However, if your net income is $56,000 and your medical expenses are $2,000, the amount that is eligible for a non-refundable tax credit would be $2,000 minus $1,728 (3% of $56,000), or $272.

Who can claim medical expenses?

Medical expenses can be claimed for yourself, your spouse, same-sex or common-law partner, your children, your partners' children or grandchildren if they depended on you for support during the tax year. Similarly, parents, grandparents, siblings, uncles, aunts, nieces or nephews who live in Canada at any time during the year and depended on you for financial support may also qualify. The calculation for the latter categories is fairly complex and often you don't receive any benefit anyway—a good reason to seek professional advice if this applies to you.

You can make a claim for medical expenses paid in any 12-month period that ended during the taxation year. In some cases, it may result in a larger claim to take a 12-month period, for example, that goes from July 1 of one year to June 30 of the next. In most cases, an amount can be claimed even if it is for expenses paid outside Canada if treatment was not available in Canada or if the illness or disabling event occurred outside Canada.

What medical expenses can be claimed?

Medical expenses cannot be claimed for any amounts that have been reimbursed or are eligible to be reimbursed by an extended health plan or other source. However, you can claim the difference between what you paid and any reimbursement you received.

The list of allowable medical expenses is very detailed and available on the CCRA Web site. Remember that not just payments to a medical doctor or for direct medical treatment qualify. For example, payments to a dentist, psychotherapist, physiotherapist, naturopath, homeopath, chiropractor, and other registered health practitioners also qualify.

Specific expenses

The following expenses can be specifically claimed for people with disabilities:

- Payments for artificial limbs, wheelchairs, crutches, hearing aids or personal assistive listening devices, prescription glasses, contact lenses, dentures, pacemakers, prescription drugs, and certain prescription medical devices
- Therapy that has been prescribed and supervised by a doctor, a psychologist or an occupational therapist

- Expenses relating to guide dogs, hearing ear, and other working animals
- Twenty per cent of the cost of a van that has been adapted (or is adapted within 6 months of purchase) to transport a person who uses a wheelchair to a limit of $5,000 (For residents of Ontario, the provincial limit is $5,135.)
- Travel expenses. If medical treatment is not available locally. The person with the disability may be eligible to claim expenses for treatment somewhere else.
- Reasonable cost of altering the driveway of the main residence of an individual with a severe and prolonged mobility impairment, to allow easier access to a bus
- Building and renovating costs on a residence for a person who has a severe and prolonged mobility impairment or who lacks normal physical development, where changes are needed to a home in order to give the person access or in order to allow them to be more mobile and functional within the home. These costs include buying and installing outdoor or indoor ramps, enlarging doors and hallways, lowering kitchen or bathroom cabinets.
- Reasonable moving expenses (which have not been claimed as moving expenses on anyone else's return) to move a person who has a severe and prolonged mobility impairment or who lacks normal physical development to housing that is more accessible to the individual or in which the individual is more mobile or functional, to a limit of $2,000 (For residents of Ontario the limit is $2,054.)
- Amount paid for the taxpayer or a relative to learn to care for a relative who has a mental or physical infirmity and who is in the taxpayer's household or is dependent on that taxpayer for support

- Fees paid to a group home, assuming nobody has claimed it as an attendant or institutional care medical expense, a childcare expense or an attendant care expense
- Amounts paid for attendant care or care in an institution for people who do not qualify for the disability amount. The taxpayer with a disability can claim only amounts paid for an attendant who was not the taxpayer's spouse or same-sex or common-law partner and who was over the age of 18. Privately hired attendants will usually be considered to be employees.
- Tutoring and talking textbooks certified as necessary by a medical practitioner because of the person's learning disability or mental impairment. Talking textbooks may also be claimed for a person who has a perceptual disability and is enrolled in an educational institution in Canada.

The following table outlines eligible medical expenses only for people with disabilities who *do not* qualify for the disability tax credit.

Claimable Medical Expenses for People who Do Not Qualify for the Disability Tax Credit

Condition	Claimable medical expense
A mental or physical infirmity, such that the person is likely to be dependent on others for his or her personal needs and care for the long term, and needs a full-time attendant, as certified in a letter from a medical practitioner	Amounts paid for full-time care by an attendant in a self-contained domestic establishment
A lack of normal mental capacity, such that the person is, and will continue to be, dependent on others for his or her personal needs and care, as certified in a letter from a medical practitioner	Amounts paid for full-time care in a nursing home

Condition	Claimable medical expense
A mental or physical handicap (including any resulting behavioural problems and learning disabilities), as certified in a letter from a medical practitioner or another appropriately qualified individual, confirming the person's need for the equipment, facilities, or personnel available in an establishment operated for the person's handicap	Amounts paid for full- or part-time care (including training) in the school, institution, nursing home, or other establishment that has the equipment, facilities, or personnel needed by people with a certain handicap

Chart, page 9 "Information Concerning people with Disabilities" CCRA Web site

Since several provinces now apply a different calculation for these credits, it is important to check with a competent tax professional, especially if the person with the disability has a spouse or is a dependent of someone else. When medical expenses are very high, and/or when the person with a disability has significantly lower income, it may be better, in fact, to claim some or all of the credits on the tax return of the supporting person who has the higher income. This requires calculating various scenarios to determine who should claim the tax credits.

Refundable medical expense supplement

A *refundable* medical expense supplement is also payable to working individuals with low *earned* income and high medical expenses. The calculation is fairly complex, but in 2002 taxpayers with earned income under $20,296 qualified for this credit. *Refundable* means that if you do not owe tax, this amount can be refunded to you. Regular medical tax credit claims are non-refundable credits.

Attendant Care Expenses

Some attendant care expenses can be claimed as medical expenses when the person may *not* be eligible for the disability tax credit. (See the preceding chart.)

There are different rules that apply in cases where the person *is* eligible for the disability tax credit. The person with the disability must be the taxpayer, their spouse or a dependent. The expenses that fall under this category are as follows:

- Attendant care
- Care in a nursing home, a school, or an institution.

An attendant must be over the age of 18 and cannot be a spouse, common-law, or same-sex partner. An attendant who is hired privately will likely be considered an employee, which means that the employer (the person with the disability or his or her representative), must register with CCRA and take payroll deductions for income tax, Canada Pension Plan and Employment Insurance premiums, and usually for Workers' Compensation, too.

Tip: Attendant care payments cannot be claimed both as a medical expense and as an attendant care expense.

People with disabilities who receive attendant care or are residents of nursing homes or other residential care facilities have two options:

Option 1
- You can claim medical expenses for full-time or part-time care of up to $10,000 ($20,000 in the year of death). Again, the provincial amounts vary.
- You can claim the disability tax credit and transfer any unused portion to a spouse or other supporting person.
- You can claim personal attendant care expenses that allowed the claimant to work, go to school, or conduct research.

Option 2

- You can claim *all* full-time or part-time care as medical expenses.
- You *cannot* claim the amount for the disability tax credit, nor can anyone else claim the disability amount on behalf of the person with the disability.
- You can claim personal attendant care expenses that allowed the claimant to work, go to school, or conduct research.

Working out which is the best option, bearing in mind the ramifications and the impact on other areas of the tax return, requires expert tax advice.

These rules are fairly complex, and, as is the case with much of the Income Tax Act, they are often revised or reinterpreted.

In many cases, people with disabilities are unable to benefit from many of these deductions because their taxable incomes are so low—they may be receiving only provincial disability benefits or CPP disability payments or non-taxable private disability insurance payments.

Childcare expenses

The normal childcare expense deduction for a child under the age of 7 is $7,000 per year. However, this amount is increased to $10,000 per year if there is a child under the age of 7 for whom the disability tax credit can be claimed. For parents who have children between the ages of 8 and 16 with a mental and/or physical infirmity, but no eligibility for the disability tax credit, the claim is $4,000. This assumes, of course, that all the other requirements of the childcare expense deduction are met and that the parents have, in fact, spent these amounts for childcare.

Normally, the spouse with the lower net income must claim the childcare expense deduction. However, there are special situations in which the supporting person with the higher net income is permitted to claim the childcare expense deduction. One of these is if the lower-income spouse was confined to bed, had to use a wheelchair for mobility, or was a patient in a hospital because of a mental or physical infirmity and was incapable of caring for their children for at least 2 consecutive weeks. To meet this requirement, you must have a letter from the attending physician stating the nature and duration of the infirmity.

The second situation is if the lower-income spouse is incapable of caring for children for a long, indefinite period of time due to a physical or mental disability. Again you must have a statement from the attending physician.

Although both the examples given above relate to very specific situations, remember that these options may be available in certain circumstances. The assumption in the Income Tax Act is that using a wheelchair, for example, means that the income of the person with the disability is lower than that of a spouse without a disability. Of course, this is not always the case.

Tuition and education amount

Tuition fees paid for post-secondary education are claimable for tax credits for all taxpayers as long as certain conditions are met. There is an additional *education amount* available assuming the person has a form T2202 from the educational institution. As long as people with disabilities are *enrolled* as full-time students, they may claim the amount of $400 per month, even if they could *attend* only on a part-time basis because of a mental or physical impairment. If the person with a disability is already eligible for the disability tax credit, no further certification is required; but if the person is not eligible for the disability tax credit, a qualified professional has to certify part 3 of form T2202.

A portion of the tuition and education amounts that cannot be used by the taxpayer may be transferred to another supporting person such as the spouse, parent, or grandparent, or carried forward to a future year.

Other amounts

There are various other amounts that taxpayers supporting people with disabilities may be able to claim, in addition to transferred medical expenses, tuition and education amounts, and the disability tax credit.

Amount for an eligible dependent (formerly *equivalent-to-spouse amount*) may be claimed by a single, widowed, divorced, or separated taxpayer for a related person who is not a spouse or common-law spouse and who has a net income below $7,131 (in 2002). If the income is below $649 the full claim is $6,482. Between $649 and $7,131, the credit is pro-rated. To qualify, the taxpayer must support the dependent and the dependent must live in the same home as the taxpayer. There is no requirement for disability.

Amount for infirm dependent age 18 or older requires a doctor's letter and applies to you or your spouse's child, grandchild, parent, grandparent, brother, sister, aunt, uncle, niece, or nephew who was a Canadian resident on December 31, and who is physically or mentally infirm. The maximum claim is $3,605. There is no claim if the dependent has net income over $8,720 (in 2002). The amount of claim will be reduced by any claim for an eligible dependent. (See above.) The dependent does not need to reside with the taxpayer in order to claim this credit.

Caregiver amount is a credit for taxpayers who are taking care of infirm dependents. The dependent must be over 18 if a child or over 65 if a parent or grandparent and must live with the taxpayer. This amount can be claimed in addition to the *amount for an eligible dependent*, but the caregiver credit will be reduced by the amount of any claim under *eligible dependent credit*. The maximum caregiver credit available was $3,605 in 2002 reduced by the dependent's net income above $12,312 (in 2002). Once the dependent's net income reaches $15,917, no credit is available.

Federal excise gasoline tax refund program

To recognize the fact that Canadians with severe mobility impairments are unable to use public transportation safely in many areas, the federal government allows for a refund of part of the federal excise tax on gasoline purchases. An information sheet is available at local CCRA tax services offices, or you can call 1-877-432-5472.

GST/HST exemptions

People with disabilities do not pay GST on the following goods and services:

- Health care services including government-funded homemaking services
- Personal care and supervision programs
- Meals-on-wheels and similar programs
- Medical devices, including incontinence products, and clothing that is specially designed for use by people with a disability upon written orders of a medical practitioner
- Recreational programs offered by a public sector body to people with disabilities

In addition, there is a rebate of GST/HST for the purchase of a motor vehicle that has already been equipped and adapted for use by a person with a wheelchair. Most of these products or services are purchased from suppliers familiar with both federal and provincial tax rules. These suppliers will not usually include GST charges on their invoices.

SOURCES OF INFORMATION

Information on all these tax matters can be obtained from *Canada Customs & Revenue Agency* or by visiting the Web site at: www.ccra-adrc.gc.ca. See the blue pages of your local telephone directory for the location and phone numbers of CCRA offices in your area.

CHAPTER 12

WHEN CAN YOU SUE?

Readers are cautioned that the information below is of a general nature only and is not designed to provide legal advice. Rather it is intended to explain how the legal system works for people with disabilities. Injured persons who feel they may have legal claims should contact a lawyer. Information on how to find and choose a lawyer is included in this chapter.

A glossary of some of the legal terms can be found at the end of this chapter.

How are Claims for Compensation Settled?

In addition to restraints on the right to sue in motor vehicle or personal injury cases, the various provincial workers' compensation plans across the country also restrict the right to sue for compensation. (See Chapter 9, "Workers' Compensation" for details on compensation for workplace injuries).

When claims for compensation arise, they are settled through two main processes:

- The accident benefit system, which is restrictive; benefits are set out by statute.
- The tort system, which is broader and proceeds through a civil court process; it is more expensive and time-consuming.

The *tort* system, which applies in all provinces except Quebec, is based on the English Common Law that has, over the centuries, set parameters for the interpretation of claims by the courts. A tort is a breach of duty for which damages can be obtained in civil court. There must be a violation of a duty owing to the *plaintiff* (person injured) by the *defendant* (person being sued). Types of tort action related to disability include, but are not limited to, slip and falls and medical malpractice, as

195

well as motor vehicle accident claims. An injured person
using the court system has to sue the *tort feasor* (person
or party that the injured person claims has caused
damage to him or her, and is therefore liable to pay
compensation for that injury). This can take many years
in court, during which time the injured person has no
source of income and no means to pay for treatment or
rehabilitation costs until the court rules on a damage
award.

In contrast, payments to an automobile accident
claimant ideally start fairly soon after the accident. In
Ontario, and some other provinces, there is still the
right to sue for damages under motor vehicle accident
benefit plans.

Quebec has a provision in its civil code that permits
lawsuits for compensation for breach of duty (delict).

THE ACCIDENT BENEFIT SYSTEM — MOTOR VEHICLE ACCIDENT CLAIMS

The 2002 edition of "Facts of the General Insurance
Industry in Canada," states:

Automobile liability insurance for private passenger
and commercial vehicles is mandatory throughout
Canada. This provides financial protection if
policyholders are held liable for injury or loss
sustained by others arising from the operation of their
vehicles. Many provinces have implemented so-called
'no-fault' schemes whereby accident victims,
regardless of fault, may claim compensation from
their own insurers for injuries. These plans range
from 'pure no-fault' in Quebec and Manitoba to
'threshold no-fault' in Ontario, 'modified pure no-
fault' in Saskatchewan and more rudimentary plans
elsewhere.

Generally, the higher the 'no-fault' threshold, the
less the involvement of the courts. Thresholds can be
monetary (e.g., above a specified dollar amount of

insured medical expenses) or verbal (a description of severely debilitating injuries, loss or impairment of bodily functions, etc); above these thresholds lawsuits may be permitted. In Ontario, for example, seriously injured claimants (and the personal representatives of persons killed in auto accidents) may sue for pain and suffering (provided that the threshold is met). All innocent victims may sue for lost income and other economic losses resulting from the injury in excess of their other sources of recovery for those losses.

No fault means that the right to sue in the case of a motor vehicle accident is determined by provincial legislation. The extent of the right to sue in each province is outlined in the publication "Facts" (as above) and on the Insurance Bureau of Canada Web site www.ibc.ca. The publication and the Web site also outline provincial standards for:

- Compulsory minimum third party liability
- Medical payments
- Funeral expense benefits
- Disability income benefits
- Death benefits
- Right to sue for pain and suffering or economic loss in excess of no-fault benefits
- Administration of plans

Motor vehicle accident claims are handled in various ways from province to province and from state to state in the United States. Some provinces and states have completely no-fault benefit systems. Others have a tort system, whereas others have a combination of the two. As a result of escalating insurance premiums in many provinces, limitations on claims are likely to become more prevalent in the next few years.

The Ontario Accident Benefits System for Motor Vehicle Accidents

Space does not permit coverage of all motor vehicle accident benefits systems. The situation in Ontario is given as an example. Check the Insurance Bureau of Canada Web site www.ibc.ca for more information on your own province's system.

What benefits are available?

In Ontario, accident benefits are provided under legislation. If a person injured in a motor vehicle accident is out of work as a result of an accident, they may claim certain benefits, such as:

- Income replacement—that is, lost wages or income from self-employment
- Medical rehabilitation and treatment
- Housekeeping
- Dependent care
- Attendant care
- Assessment costs
- Other benefits—including an amount for spouses and dependents

In the case of extended health benefits such as physiotherapy, chiropractic, and other rehabilitation treatments, the *first payor* (the insurance company that pays out first), is any private or group insurance the injured person may have. Claims for rehabilitation and treatment from the auto insurer are all *secondary* payments. This means that if you have an extended health benefits policy, you must claim under that policy first. Once you have used up benefits under the extended health policy, the auto insurer will cover the rest if they approve the treatment plan.

The accident benefit system in Ontario does *not* allow claims for *pain and suffering*, normally referred to as *general damages*. To claim for pain and suffering, a claimant must launch a tort claim. (See section on Tort Claims.)

If you are a claimant in a motor vehicle accident, you can go after both accident benefits *and* a tort claim. If you forgo (do not take) accident benefits *before* mediation, you may lose accident benefits altogether. Or you may forgo the accident benefits *after* mediation but then claim both tort and accident benefits together.

Catastrophic injury claims

If the injury is defined as *catastrophic*, which typically means that the injured person has been unconscious, in a coma, and/or totally disabled, then benefits may be payable beyond 104 weeks and may be payable indefinitely. The maximum claim for rehabilitation increases to $1 million over 10 years from $100,000 in a non-catastrophic situation. Attendant care coverage increases to lifetime coverage from a maximum of 2 years.

How are benefits calculated?

Benefits payable under the accident benefits system depend on the prior earnings of the person injured. For a salaried employee in Ontario, it is 80% of his or her net weekly income before the accident up to a maximum of $400 per week. This income benefit is tax-free. This amount is not indexed to inflation and is not adjusted. The maximum payment period is 2 years or 104 weeks, but a policyholder can pay additional automobile insurance premiums and increase this amount to $600, $800 or $1,000 per week, assuming they have the prior earnings to justify this amount. The calculation of benefits for someone who is self-employed is significantly more complex and is beyond the scope of this book.

Planning tips: If you have no disability insurance, or very little disability insurance, you should consider buying additional automobile insurance benefits. In the event of an automobile accident, you will then have some income replacement available to you.

If the injured person is a student who misses schooling to the extent that tuition costs are incurred for time not at school, this amount may be recoverable. If the student is not employed, there may be no lost income claim.

There are different approaches to electing or choosing which benefits to take after a motor vehicle accident.

For example, a low-income worker injured in a car accident may be eligible for $100 per week in income replacement benefits. If that worker has young children or another person dependent upon them for care, such as a parent, he or she may elect to receive instead up to $300 per week, as long as he or she is unable to perform activities involved in caregiving. This amount would be received in order to pay someone else to take over or assist in the caregiving role.

People who are injured in motor vehicle accidents should obtain the advice of a lawyer as soon as possible. They should not try to represent themselves, as the area of law involving accident benefits and tort are complex. Although paralegals will charge less than lawyers, they may also be less inclined to pursue the case beyond the first level of mediation if they are not going to get significantly more money for their time. Not all paralegals carry liability insurance because it is not a regulated profession.

✔ **Warning:** People involved in car accidents should be very wary of tow truck operators handing out business cards for paralegals or lawyers specializing in personal injury claims or rehabilitation centres. "Kickbacks" are not uncommon. Nor is it uncommon for people to start getting rehabilitation without having approval for payment from the insurance company, but the insurance company is entitled to refuse the claim. Phone your automobile insurance carrier to ask what procedure they want you to follow. Then contact a lawyer if needed.

Mistakes made in motor vehicle accident benefit claims:

- Not retaining a lawyer
- Not getting appropriate legal advice
- Not keeping complete records and documenting everything. The types of documentation required include:
  — Drug receipts
  — Name, date, and place of doctor's visits. Make sure you get the name of the doctor who treated you if you went to a walk-in clinic or to an emergency room.
  — Rehabilitation costs
  — If someone stays home to take care of the injured person, document all incurred expenses, including evidence of the number of hours, who was doing what, where, why, and when. In other words, record as much detail as possible. This can cover attendant care for the activities of daily living and housework.
  — In Ontario, you will require a Form 1 that records the treatment plan and cost breakdown.
  — Remember to claim for such items as eyeglasses that may have been broken in the accident, hearing aids and any clothing that was damaged. Make sure you retain receipts for any out-of-pocket expenditures in this area.

In Ontario, accident benefits cover 15 treatments over 6 weeks for physiotherapy and chiropractic adjustments *with a treatment plan*. A treatment plan is normally drawn up by the medical practitioner treating the patient, often a physiotherapist or chiropractor. If there is no treatment plan, the insurance company may be within its rights to refuse to pay the benefits.

If the treatment plan is turned down by the insurer, the claimant may need to go to a *Disability Assessment Centre* (DAC). There can be different assessment centres for different needs. If the claimant doesn't go to a DAC, they could be on the hook financially for treatment if the insurance company turns down their claim. In order to appeal this decision, the claimant has to go to an adjudicator or judge. If the claimant loses at appeal then they are going to have to pay for the treatment out of their own pocket.

✔ Warning: There are a lot of rip-offs in this area. An unethical rehabilitation centre may offer to provide transportation by taxicab to and from treatment—but this is added to the bill! For example, for a claimant living in Toronto who suffers mild whiplash, an insurer is unlikely to agree to pay for taxis to and from physiotherapy when the claimant could take public transit. Be advised: "If it looks too good to be true, it probably is". In other words, do not sign up for anything without checking with your insurer first and having their agreement to pay the costs.

If you are hurt on a bus, at least in Ontario, it is considered a motor vehicle accident and you can claim through the accident benefits system. But the subway is not a motor vehicle!

If you are injured in any way in a motor vehicle accident when you are not the driver, but you have automobile insurance coverage, you must still call your own insurance carrier first, since all claims go through them. This will *not* affect your own automobile insurance rates. This applies even if you are a pedestrian, a passenger on a bus, or are injured by a passing car, motorcycle, or truck. If however, you have no automobile insurance, and nobody in the immediate household has automobile insurance, then the first claim is against the person who hit you. For this reason, it is still *very important* that the injured person obtain insurance information from the person who hit them. If this is not possible, then the licence number of the vehicle will help.

The insurance company is obligated to explain all benefits to which the injured person is entitled in a way that they can understand. This includes having an interpreter provided by the insurance company if necessary.

Does it matter where the accident took place?

Normally, the province or state where the accident took place is the jurisdiction whose rules apply in a particular circumstance. However, case law is always evolving in this area. For example, in a situation where two Ontario residents in separate cars are involved in an accident in Florida or another tort state, the plaintiff (injured party) would likely prefer to sue under Florida law (a tort state) because tort settlements in the United States are usually significantly higher than they are in Canada. The defendant's insurance company, on the other hand, would prefer that Ontario law apply, since the cost to them would be significantly lower.

Disputes

It is very important to be represented if there are any disputes as to the claim. Usually, disputes arise because the insurance company considers that the claimant is cured, and the claimant disagrees. In Ontario, the claimant then applies for mediation. At this stage, the injured claimant is on one side and the insurance company is on the other. At this point it becomes an adversarial system. There is a *pre-hearing*, and if the claim is not resolved at this point, it goes to an *arbitration hearing*.

The victim of a motor vehicle accident in Ontario can choose either to go to court or to arbitration. Through the courts, it may take several years to settle a claim. The arbitration process starts within a few months. In addition, the court system is much more stressful for the victim.

The whole point of the motor vehicle accident benefits system in Canada is to provide timely payment of some benefits to a person who has been disabled in a motor vehicle accident, rather than having that person wait for what may amount to several years for the court system to settle a claim.

Deductibles

There is a $15,000 deductible from the amount awarded. For example, if the injury is assessed at $100,000, then $15,000 comes off the top and the claimant receives $85,000. For Family Law Act claims, there is a $7,500 deductible for each claimant. (See section later in this chapter, "Under what circumstances can you sue?", for a discussion of possible Family Law Act claims.)

Legal fees

Unless there is mediation or arbitration, the claimant pays the legal fees on accident benefits claims. Only if a case goes to mediation or arbitration are fees negotiated as part of the settlement.

What happens if the amount claimed is greater than the defendant's liability coverage?

For amounts above and beyond the defendant's insurance coverage, the plaintiff (injured person) sues the defendants personally in tort (see next section). They also name their own insurance company as a defendant under the "under insured" coverage provision. This provides coverage if the defendant has no insurance coverage or insufficient insurance coverage themselves. For example, if the defendant has $1 million of liability coverage, and the plaintiff has $1 million of coverage, but the settlement is $3 million, both insurance companies would pay out. Then the plaintiff goes after other assets that the defendant owns personally such as a house, cottage, or retirement savings.

Remember that the specifics of the accident benefit system described above reflect only the situation in Ontario. Some provinces have provincially run automobile insurance and the system is different. Ontario does not operate a separate motor vehicle insurance system, as some other provinces do, like British Columbia, for example.

THE TORT SYSTEM

What makes a tort claim?

Although most tort claims are motor vehicle related, there are other situations when a tort claim may be made. These include slip and falls and malpractice claims.

To succeed in a *motor vehicle* negligence tort claim, the injured person must have permanent and serious injury to an important bodily function, either physical or psychological, or a permanent disfigurement. The latter definition may depend to some extent on the nature of the injured person's occupation. For example, a fashion or swimsuit model with a two-inch red scar on one arm may well be considered to have suffered a disfigurement, whereas someone who is an office worker with the same scar would not. Similarly, a concert pianist with a badly broken finger may still be able to write, but not play the piano. As such, this definition can be very subjective and will take into account many factors. This type of claim can be quite substantial.

Proving permanent and serious injury in motor vehicle negligence tort claims can sometimes be problematic. In cases of psychological damage, testing will prove or disprove the claim.

In general tort claims, "pain and suffering" can take precedence over damages for injuries. The injuries do not need to be severe and permanent or even serious in order to launch a tort claim.

Under what circumstances can you sue?

The tort claim is a lawsuit where you can sue the offending party for the following:

- "Pain and suffering", normally referred to as general damages;
- That portion of lost income that is not covered by accident benefits, including future income loss.
- Loss of "care, guidance and companionship," which is brought forward by family members of the injured person under the Family Law Act
- The value of services other members of the family have rendered to the injured party

The primary person instituting the action, though, is the one with the injuries. They may sue the other party for pain and suffering, uncovered rehabilitation benefits, uncovered treatment benefits, and additional lost income. They can claim for damages to cover such items as assistive devices, wheelchairs, purchase of an accessible home, or renovations to a home to make it accessible, or provision of a wheelchair accessible van.

After an injury...

Injuries are not always felt immediately after an accident and, as is the case with some soft tissue injuries, it may take time before the full impact of the injury becomes evident. If a person is injured in a motor vehicle accident and the injury is orthopaedic (i.e., injury to muscles or bones), it is likely that the injured person will notice right away. If an injured person is unconscious, or is deemed to be rendered unconscious, there is the possibility of head injury and consequently the possibility of brain damage. The level of unconsciousness and length of time of unconsciousness will be considered. Therefore, if you have been involved in an accident and something doesn't feel quite right, you should go to your family physician or an emergency room as soon as possible.

The injured person must be very specific about what the complaints are and what doesn't feel right so that proper notes are kept, should evidence be needed at a later date. If the family physician cannot make a complete diagnosis, the patient may be referred to a specialist and for follow-up diagnostic testing.

In other tort claims, such as slip and falls or medical malpractice, the injured party must show damages and negative outcomes and that the party being sued owed a duty of care and was negligent in breaching it. There is no threshold as to the amount of damages that may be claimed.

Who can you sue?

To determine whom the plaintiff can name in the lawsuit, the question that must be answered is "Who owes the *duty of care*?" In other words, who can reasonably be held responsible for the conditions of the injury? If a claimant has one injury that meets the threshold, there is a claim for all other injuries even if the other injuries on their own would not meet the threshold for injuries (i.e., permanent and serious).

Some examples of possible claims

- After a snowstorm, snow on the ground melts and then freezes, forming a sheet of ice. The homeowner does nothing about it despite a duty to take care. If an invited visitor falls and injures him or herself, the homeowner can be sued. If the homeowner had hired a snow removal contractor, the contractor could be sued as a third party.

- Someone drops a taco with cheese sauce in the food court of a mall, and another person slips and falls and injures him or herself. The store, the mall, and the maintenance company could all be sued if they have been careless in failing to clean up when it was their duty to do so.

Payment for injuries incurred as a result of risky pastimes like water-skiing or horseback riding depend on the specifics of the situation. For example, a parent takes his child to a fair, pays to have a ride on a horse, and the horse does something unexpected that results in the child breaking a bone. Unless the parent signed a very explicit waiver ahead of time, there would be a claim. On the other hand, if a person is an avid horseback rider, is part of an equestrian group, owns the horse, rents space at a stable, and the horse does something to that person, there is unlikely to be a claim.

There are always atypical claims. For instance, a woman was sitting on a bench in a mall when a maintenance man came through with a pushcart piled high with boxes of merchandise. A box fell off the top and hit her on the head. She was 8 months' pregnant at the time and became an emotional invalid after that. The claim was settled for a substantial amount.

These are reasons why it is important not to settle these cases too quickly. You want to have a very secure prognosis before any realistic settlement is made. This involves getting several different assessments over a period of time so that you can judge the likely improvement over time. This is particularly true of closed-head injuries.

Some situations lend themselves to a definitive prognosis more easily than others. For example, a broken bone that heals well is less traumatic than a case where hardware, that will have to be removed later, is put into the bone to assist mending. In the latter case, there may be a greater likelihood of arthritis developing later on. Joint injuries, in general, are usually more serious because of the likelihood of arthritis developing in the joint.

Legal fees

All lawyers need instructions from the client and these are contained in a contract called a *retainer*. The retainer will spell out what the fee structure is.

In Ontario, legal fees in tort cases may be a percentage of the ultimate recovered amount. If the case is resolved before going to court, then the legal fees are normally a part of the negotiations. If the case goes to court, and if the plaintiff (claimant) is successful, then there can be costs awarded against the defendants. This will not be equal to all of the legal fees, but can form part of them.

Most insurance and personal injury lawyers will explain what their hourly rate is. Based on experience, the fees usually work out to be 15% to 33% of the amount of the settlement. There should be a correlation between the number of documented hours the lawyer puts in and the final billing. This can be adjusted depending on the complexity of the case. Of course, the longer the case goes on, the higher the billing will be. If the case goes to the eve of trial, there may be a premium for that and the percentage is likely to be closer to the 33% range or even higher, whereas if it were settled at an earlier stage, such as at discovery, it would be lower.

In Ontario, the Law Society of Upper Canada has recently allowed claimants to enter into contingency fee arrangements with their lawyers, except in criminal and family law matters. A contingency fee ties the fee the lawyer charges to the outcome of the case so that if the client wins, the client pays the lawyer either a percentage or other agreed-upon amount of the settlement. If the client loses, the client doesn't pay. The lawyer therefore accepts the risk of not being paid when accepting a contingency fee case.

When lawyers consider taking on a personal injury case, they will determine whether there is any value in taking on that particular case. In other words, is there a good chance they can get a good settlement for their client? If they think it's a good case, they may agree to fund it to get the relevant medical assessments and other assessments done, which can be quite expensive. Not until the end of the case will the lawyer be compensated. The lawyer is carrying the claimant financially for all costs until the case is settled, which is often several years. If it is a problematic case, for example where there are liability issues, lawyers will probably tell the client that they are not agreeable to funding the expenses for the client, and that they will take the case only with a retainer paid upfront to cover the medical assessments and other disbursements.

When are most cases settled?

The vast majority of cases get settled before trial. There are numerous factors that influence pre-trial settlements. Usually, the more significant the injury, the easier the claim is to settle. It is usually a question of the insurer coming up with more money rather than arguing about the facts of the case. It is the less obvious cases, when there are more likely to be accusations of malingering, that drag on and may ultimately end up in court. In some cases, the arguments may be based on who is at fault, or whether the plaintiff is or is not totally disabled.

The appropriate medical assessments must be done in order to assess the amount of damages to claim. The motivations of the lawyers can affect the outcome and the speed of the settlement. One lawyer who requests anonymity comments:

> "Unfortunately, there are some lawyers who just want to hang on to an insurance file for as long as possible so that they can bill as many hours as possible in a particular case. Sometimes the client's personality can affect the outcome of the case or the length of time it takes to settle, especially when it is someone with moderate injuries who thinks that they are entitled to a higher settlement amount."

Which cases typically go to trial?

Cases that go to trial are often ones when there is the possibility of a new interpretation of the law, or when the *jurisprudence* (previous decisions) in several other important jurisdictions is leaning one way, while in the province where the new case is being heard, jurisprudence is leaning in another. Often, these cases end up going to appeal.

There can be conflicting arguments for liability from the plaintiffs' side and the defendants' side. Degrees of fault and contributory negligence can become issues. At a trial, the credibility of witnesses on each side, who may each attest to a different version of what happened, will be weighed up by the court, to try and come up with a true sequence of events. Each side may also offer different assessments of the damages involved.

Case history:

A young plaintiff was unconscious at the scene of the accident, suffered brain injury, and was away from school for several months recovering. She went back to school, but required a tutor for the rest of public school and still did very well. She was an A+ student before her accident. After her accident she was a B+/A student. She went on and got her Bachelor of Science degree, again with the help of a tutor right through university. She wanted to go into a professional school—and at this point she started to have difficulties, even with the help of a tutor. Finding a tutor at that level also became difficult. It became clear that she was going to have a very difficult time obtaining a professional degree.

This is one of the arguments for not settling lawsuits too quickly, as it is often only after a period of time has elapsed that the true long term impact of damages can be properly assessed. In the case described above, not only was there a claim for the tutoring, there was also a claim for lost earnings potential.

Where do you find a lawyer to handle a disability or personal injury/motor vehicle accident claim?

When looking for a lawyer to act for you, remember that disability claims are different from personal injury claims, and that motor vehicle claims are different from claims for slips and falls. Therefore, it is important to:

- Look for a lawyer who has experience in your particular type of claim
- Look for lawyer who has been practising for some time and is aware of the law in the specific area, because the laws are always changing
- Ask how much the lawyer charges, since fees should be discussed right at the beginning. Fee schedules should be put in writing so that there is no misunderstanding as to how compensation is to be calculated.

In most provinces, you can get one half hour of free legal consultation, likely over the phone. Start with referrals from your provincial Law Society, which will direct you to accident benefit, personal injury, or disability insurance lawyers in your area. The very best referral is from someone who has had a similar experience and was pleased with his or her lawyer.

What are the maximum claims awarded by the courts?

The major factors that influence the amount of damages are as follows:

- Type of injury
- Age of victim
- Occupation of victim
- Long term prognosis

Most disability related cases are settled before trial and damages or settlement awards are not recorded. For example, a settlement for a broken leg can range from $25,000 to $125,000 depending on the type of break, whether a metal plate and screws have to be put into the leg, whether the plate may have to be removed later, and whether there is the possibility of arthritis developing in the future.

In terms of lost income, much depends on how much earned income the person was making before they became disabled. The amount can be puny or astronomical.

For example, in the case of a Chief Executive Officer of a major corporation making a high salary with large year-end bonuses who is unable to work as a result of a disability caused by an accident, the settlement is likely to be in the millions of dollars. If the injured person has quadriplegia, uses a wheelchair and needs constant care, future care claims can again run into the millions of dollars. Even so, compared with what is awarded in the United States, claim amounts in Canada are relatively low.

In the case of someone who can be held partially to blame for the injury sustained, damages awarded and the apportionment of blame is different from the case of someone who has not engaged in any risky behaviour or cannot be held to be partially responsible for their injury.

For example, someone who got into an automobile knowing that the driver was intoxicated, and was injured in a resulting accident when the driver was at fault, might be held to be partly to blame for the injuries suffered. Damages would be expected to be lower than in a case with the same injury when the driver was not intoxicated and had a good driving record.

What is the time frame within which a tort claim must be made?

In motor vehicle accidents, the time frame for making a claim is 2 years from the date you ought to have known you suffered injuries from the motor vehicle accident. Sometimes there are latent injuries that are not readily apparent at the time of the accident. In most cases, it is 2 years from the date of the accident.

With slip and falls, dog bites, and other personal injury claims, the time limit is usually 6 years from the date of the incident.

To be on the safe side, you should see a lawyer immediately if you have suffered any substantial injury. As the claimant, you should not be concerned about time periods; that is something for the lawyer to handle. The general rule is, if in doubt, contact a lawyer and get a legal opinion in the case of any injury.

Checklist for all personal injury and accident situations

- ✔ Report the accident to the police if it is a motor vehicle accident
- ✔ Call your insurance company immediately with all details
- ✔ See a doctor or get hospital treatment immediately to get checked over. Keep notes as to who examined you and what they said.
- ✔ Find a lawyer who specializes in the area of your potential claim

In all potential claims situations:

- ✔ Keep accurate records from the time of the incident. (A diary is a good idea.)
- ✔ Save all receipts for medication, therapy and other injury-related supplies.
- ✔ Record all visits to doctors, including date and time, name address, phone number and notes about the visit.
- ✔ Remember to include receipts for replacement clothes, eyeglasses, shoes or any other items damaged in the event.

Note: At press time, changes to Ontario regulations were about to be brought into law. They would open up tort remedies for individuals who had serious, but not catastrophic injuries. New treatment protocols are also to be introduced.

SOURCES OF INFORMATION

The Insurance Bureau of Canada
  151 Yonge St., Toronto, Ontario M5C 2W7 (416) 362-2031
  www.ibc.ca
This is the national organization of general insurers (property
  and casualty insurers). They also have a dispute resolution
  service called The General Insurance OmbudService (GIO).
  (For Ontario disputes, go to the Financial Services
  Commission of Ontario).
Law Society of Upper Canada www.lsuc.on.ca

GLOSSARY

Contingency Fee: The amount of compensation paid to the
  lawyer is related to the degree of success achieved in the
  proceedings. Provincial Law Societies regulate this area.
Defendant: The person being sued or defending the action
Duty of Care: An obligation to be careful
First Payor: The insurance company that pays benefits first
Plaintiff: The injured party, the person suing
Tort: Private or civil wrong or injury; a breach of duty for
  which damages can be obtained in civil court
Tort feasor: A wrong doer; one who is guilty of a tort

CHAPTER 13

LEGAL SETTLEMENT OPTIONS FOR PERSONAL INJURY CLAIMS

If legal action is taken on behalf of a person who sustains injury as a result of a motor vehicle accident or personal injury claim or as a result of malpractice and the claim is successful, then the court will mandate payment to the individual with a disability.

A successful claim or lawsuit means that the person with the disability is awarded a *settlement* or sum of cash to compensate for the disability. There are two main ways that funds are paid out:

- Structured settlements
- Lump sum

There are advantages and disadvantages to both types of payout. But the most important fact to note is that an American study showed that within *2 months* of receiving a significant monetary windfall as a lump sum, such as lottery winnings, a large inheritance or personal injury award, about 25% of recipients had nothing left. At the end of the first year, 50% had nothing left. At the end of 2 years, 70% had nothing left. And at the end of 5 years, 90% had nothing left.

STRUCTURED SETTLEMENTS

Instead of a one-time, lump-sum payment, a structured settlement is one in which the recipient receives an income over a period of time. This is negotiated, usually through a lawyer, for the recipient or on his/her behalf by a spouse, parents, or other family members. The structured settlement functions like an annuity in that the insurance company responsible for the settlement purchases an annuity from a federally regulated life insurance company. The insurance company guarantees periodic payments (usually monthly) to the recipient for the remainder of the recipient's life, or for a specified number of years (for example, 10 or 15 years).

How Do Structured Settlements Work?

Each payment from a structured settlement, is a combination of capital and interest, just like an annuity. But all of it is received tax–free, whereas a normal annuity will have a taxable component to it. Some key points to remember are:

- The amount of payment cannot be changed once the settlement agreement has been set up.
- Payments cannot be seized in the event of bankruptcy.
- Payments are not subject to Family Law Act calculations or division.
- Payments can be received monthly, quarterly, semi-annually, or annually.
- Payments may be indexed to the Consumer Price Index (CPI) and adjusted once a year. (There is no cap on a CPI-linked settlement, but payments will not decrease during a time of deflation.)
- The recipient can choose to receive lump-sum amounts at specific future dates as part of the settlement, if negotiated in the original agreement. (For example, the individual may need a new van or wheelchair every 10 years and would receive lump sums to cover those expenses.)
- If the beneficiary is a young person requiring the care of parents, the settlement may be structured so that, at the point when the parents can no longer care for their child, income from the structured settlement increases to cover the cost of hiring caregivers.
- There can be a *guarantee period* that protects the recipient's estate. That is, there could be a minimum 25 years of payments that must be paid

out, to a spouse or another named beneficiary, tax-free, regardless of how long the recipient lives. If the recipient has, or may have, dependents or a spouse, these guarantees can be very useful. There is a cost to include such guarantees in a structured settlement.

- Depending upon the nature of the disability, it may be possible for the recipient to receive a higher monthly payment if their life expectancy is actuarially deemed to be reduced. This is called an *impairment rating*. (The person will not necessarily die sooner, but it is possible. Therefore, the insurance company bets that it will not have to pay out for as long a period of time.)

Solvency and Other Guarantees on Structured Settlements

There are three types of guarantees that apply to structured settlements:

✔ The issuing life insurance company must be a federally registered Canadian life insurance company with 100 years or more of continuous operation. It must have assets in excess of $25 billion dollars. It must be highly rated, have excellent financial security, and have significantly more assets than liabilities. This is to ensure that the chance of the insurance company defaulting on its obligations is virtually none.

✔ The Canadian Life and Health Insurance Compensation Corporation (CompCorp) guarantees up to $2,000 per month in payments in the event that the life insurance company defaults or goes bankrupt.

✔ The original casualty insurance company (whether automobile, home or other liability insurance company that had to pay out the settlement,) remains liable for payments to the recipient with a disability *even if* the life insurance company defaults, and the CompCorp coverage is insufficient to meet the obligations to the recipient. In other words, if the life insurance company paying out the structured settlement goes broke, and the amount of payment is more than $2,000 per month (the amount covered by CompCorp) the original motor vehicle or other casualty insurance company is still liable and must pay benefits directly to the insured person.

How Structured Settlements are Developed

No-fault accident benefits, typically received as a result of a motor vehicle accident, can be paid out under a structured settlement. As with other structured settlements, guarantee periods can be negotiated to include payments that may go beyond the lifetime of the person with a disability. However, no-fault benefits paid monthly stop immediately upon death.

Large settlements received as a result of an accident or malpractice may have a structured settlement component as well as a lump sum. The lump sum can be used to pay legal fees, to pay off debts such as a mortgage, lines of credit, credit cards, or to purchase items such as a wheelchair accessible van, or to set up a "rainy day fund."

There is no maximum amount for a structured settlement, but the largest reported in Canada is about $6 million, the smallest, $1,000. Realistically, amounts under $100,000 do not make much economic sense as structured settlements for most adults. It is important, however, to realize that an award of $30,000 made on behalf of an 8-year-old would grow substantially over time. If the amount were paid into court, and invested by the official guardian's office, when that 8-year-old turns 18, he or she would receive the full amount. By using a structured settlement, the temptation to "blow it all" would be curtailed and his or her best interests protected long term.

More than one life insurance company may be used to meet the obligations of a structured settlement. For example, if a monthly income of $2,000 is to be paid in addition to a lump sum of say, $25,000 for a van every 5 years, then one insurance company may pay the monthly income, whereas another may be the payor for the van payment every 5 years.

Some provinces can order structured settlements to be put in place if the case comes before their courts. Ontario and Manitoba require structured settlements in certain cases. Alberta and Nova Scotia are reviewing this. Structured settlements can be ordered in British Columbia in automobile cases. In Quebec, a structured settlement is required for minor recipients (under age 18)—but the settlement is commutable (the person can receive the entire lump sum) at age 18!

Structured Settlements versus Investing Lump Sums

Critics of structured settlements say that the yield on a lump sum invested in the stock market is higher than that received through a structured settlement. Depending upon market conditions over a long period of time, that may, or may not, be a valid criticism. However, there are some things to remember:

- Income from the structured settlement is received *tax-free*. For someone in the lowest tax bracket, assuming a structured settlement investment pays interest at a rate of 5%, then a lump-sum investment (since the income is taxable) would need to earn 6.6% in order to match the 5% from the structured settlement. At a 40% tax bracket, the investment return on the lump sum would have to be 8.3% to match 5% on the structured settlement, At a 50% tax bracket, the investment return would have to be about 10%.
- By receiving taxable income, that is income from investments, the recipient may lose out on other

tax-free benefits. These may include lower provincial tax credits, child tax benefits, and GST tax credit.

- The impact of spending part of a large settlement can be significant. For example, with a lump-sum award of $750,000 designed to replace lost income for life, the recipient may decide to spend 10% ($75,000) on a fancy car—which sits in the driveway most of the time. In addition to much higher insurance, maintenance and fuel costs, the person has just spent $75,000 that was intended to replace future lost income. This means the recipient has dipped into capital at an earlier point than estimated and causes a serious likelihood of depleting capital entirely prior to death—most likely within 10 years.

Note: In the following sections we use the term *advisor* as a generic term; the Canadian Securities Administrators use the term *adviser* as a legal term to describe certain types of individuals licensed by the various provincial Securities Commissions.

LUMP-SUM PAYMENTS

A lump-sum payment is a one-time, tax-free payment that is designed to:
- Compensate the injured person for financial loss
- Compensate the injured person for pain and suffering, in some cases

Lump-sum payments may be for a small amount, say a few thousand dollars, in compensation for a relatively mild disabling event such as a broken leg. Or they may be for a large sum, perhaps into the millions of dollars, if the serious injury results in quadriplegia or brain injury, which has long term effects. It is these large settlements that must be handled carefully.

Once received, recipients must invest the payment wisely. The intention is that lump sums, invested, will generate the income stream needed to help people with disabilities maintain their living standard and provide personal care for the rest of their lives.

In practice, this often doesn't happen. There are several reasons for this:

- Most recipients do not invest funds properly because they are unable to do so because of their injury, or because they do not have the training or experience to do so.

- Some recipients follow the advice of well-meaning, but unqualified, friends and family members as to how and where the funds should be invested—to their detriment.

- Many recipients become the victims of the "casino mentality," of having "found money," and "share the wealth" with friends and family.

- The initial lump-sum payment is not taxable; income earned on the invested capital *is* taxable each year. Long term planning must cover taxes as well as income needs.

- If the investment income is less than what is needed to meet living needs, then the individual must dip into capital in order to maintain their living standards—or reduce his/her costs. Over time, the capital could run out.

- If the settlement is paid into court because the recipient of the settlement is a minor child, then at the age of majority (usually age 18 or 19 depending up on the jurisdiction), the child receives the whole lump sum. Most people at this age are not capable of effectively managing large sums of money that must fund their needs over the rest of their lives.

- Many financial advisors are not knowledgeable about the ramifications of investing such large sums of money for such a long period of time.

- Some advisors do not understand the concept and advantages of the structured settlement and urge their disabled clients to opt instead to take a lump sum.
- Often, advisors do not really take into account the fact that the person with a disability may never work again. If the person with a disability is not facing up to that possibility, it may not be communicated to the investment advisor either.
- Some advisors do not take into account the possible family law issues that can arise. In most provinces, all assets accumulated during marriage are divided on divorce, but insurance settlements are exempt from this rule. However, if a lump-sum, or part of it, is invested jointly or in the other spouse's name alone, and the couple separates/ divorces, the exemption under family law for money received as an insurance settlement may be lost. The other spouse may therefore receive half the settlement amount plus half of any increase in value. Since the settlement is intended to provide income for the person with a disability and not his/her spouse, this defeats the purpose of the insurance settlement. The person with the disability can be left impoverished.
- Some of the investment alternatives available for lump sums do not pay much income to financial advisors; commissions and/or management fees on bond investments, for example, are lower than those on stocks. People with disabilities must be very certain of the advice that they are receiving from advisors. Is the advisor acting in the best interests of the client, or in the best interests of the advisor? Reputable advisors will either decline the case and refer to another advisor, or will give the advice that best meets the client's interests, regardless of the fact that no significant income may be received by the advisor.

Investing Lump-Sum Settlements

For those individuals who do not (or cannot) select a structured settlement, the full responsibility for managing the lump sum is in their hands—or those of their attorneys or family. The biggest problem is getting responsible advice coupled with reasonable, consistent rates of return over a long period of time.

Most people are not competent to manage their own investments successfully over time. The American millionaire, Bernard Baruch, said in the early twentieth century that those who have significant assets should hire the best money managers that they could afford and then leave the investing decisions to them. The problem is that many advisors do not know how to invest for the long term; many have the short-term goal of placing people in the simplest investment format possible—usually mutual funds.

Many inexperienced advisors do not know when to advise clients to sell the mutual funds or other securities in which the client is invested. Although there is a trend in the investment sales world toward *unbundled* investment services, in which the client pays a fee for advice and a low fee on the investments chosen, many advisors still have no particular expertise in choosing investments that are suited to clients with disabilities. In most instances, that client needs investments that will preserve his or her capital and provide reasonably assured inflation-protected income.

Advisors need to understand that there are serious ramifications to investing settlements as lump sums. The need for capital safety and a secure, long term income flow is much more crucial for people with disabilities than for most of the advisor's other clients. Inappropriate investments for a person with a serious disability may mean that person will live in poverty for the rest of their lives.

It is also important for an advisor to recognize that the person with the disability may be being pressured or coerced into agreeing to invest in things that are inappropriate or that might be more to the advantage of another family member—not the person with a disability who is the client.

Obtaining appropriate investment advice and services

Finding the right advisor is not easy. Individuals with a disability or their representatives, whether family members or other holders of power of attorney, must become knowledgeable consumers of investment management.

Investment advice, portfolio management and trading in securities (including mutual funds, stocks, bonds, derivatives, investment trusts etc.) are matters regulated by the provincial Securities Commissions across Canada. The national organization for the Securities Commissions is known as the Canadian Securities Administrators.

Go to the Web site for the Canadian Securities Administrators: www.csa-acvm.ca. In addition to links to all the provincial Securities Commissions, you will find a section that is called "Choosing Your Financial Advisers." It contains subheadings such as:

- What Types of Financial Advisers Are There?
- Where Do I Start?
- What Questions Should I Ask?

The list of advisers is generic and condensed to two main types: dealers and advisers.

Dealers

Under the *dealer* category, there are many different types of service providers. In general, dealers are individuals, firms, or corporations that buy and sell securities, including mutual funds, for others, and who may give incidental advice about doing so. They may range in size from small to large, local to national. The client usually makes the final decision on each investment. But in some cases, investment dealers are permitted to exercise discretionary authority over a client's account.

Some investment dealers provide a full range of research, trading and advisory services; whereas others specialize in low-cost trading services for investors who wish to make their own investment decisions without seeking advice.

Mutual fund dealers are limited to dealing only in mutual fund securities and to providing advice that is incidental to such dealing. Some mutual fund dealers may also purchase certain securities for clients, such as guaranteed investment certificates, which are considered to be *exempt securities*. Mutual fund dealers sometimes call themselves "financial planners." Their usual method of compensation is commission fees. But as noted above, there is a trend toward "unbundling", which means that the salesperson receives a lower commission coupled with a fee for advice. Instead of basing their compensation on commissions and trailer fees, some firms charge fees based on a percentage of the client's account.

Advisers

Advisers provide advice to clients about investing in securities. There are different types of advisers. The services offered by advisers depend upon their registration category. For example, an *investment counsel* can provide you with investment advice and can manage your investment portfolio. If investment counsels are also registered as *portfolio managers*, then you can give them the discretionary authority to make investment decisions on your behalf and to implement those decisions. As part of their advisory services, portfolio managers can offer their clients separately managed accounts, pooled fund accounts and proprietary mutual funds, if the clients meet minimum investment thresholds set by the portfolio management firm.

- *Separately managed accounts* consist of individual investments such as stocks and bonds. These are normally available only above a certain dollar amount. They offer the ability to control capital gains and losses within individual taxpayer's portfolios, which can be critical to minimizing income taxes.
- *Pooled funds* are normally offered to investment counsel clients, too, and are used for smaller accounts. Operating in a similar way to mutual funds, their management fees are often lower than traditional mutual funds.
- *Proprietary mutual funds* are in-house mutual funds exclusively available to the organization's clients. Sometimes these funds are from firms outside the firm, but they are not available to the general public.

To better understand investments, see the "Sources of Information" section at the end of this chapter for recommended reading.

There is usually a minimum investment amount required before such advisers will accept an account, ranging from about $250,000 to several million dollars.

Such advisers are compensated with fees based on a percentage of assets under management, not on trading activity. As noted, they must also be licensed as investment counsellors (advisers) under provincial securities regulations. They do *not* receive commissions or trailer fees or additional fees from investment products. The fee for such investment management by investment counsellors on non-registered accounts is deductible from the recipient's taxable income.

What You Need to Know about Advice-givers

Financial planners who buy and sell securities (including mutual funds) must be licensed by the provincial Securities Commission. There is no precise definition of the terms *financial adviser* or *financial planner*—terms that are used interchangeably. Only Quebec regulates who may call themselves *financial advisers* or *financial planners*.

Those who sell insurance and related products are licensed under the various provincial Insurance Commissions. As insurance brokers, they sell insurance products, and, on the investment side, segregated funds. (Segregated funds are basically mutual funds but with special guarantees exclusive to life insurance issuers). They may also be called financial planners.

Financial planning and financial advisory services available to you can vary dramatically, depending upon who is offering the service and what these people actually do as planners or advisors.

There is not necessarily a correlation between good advice and an absence of commission-based compensation. Keep in mind that, for the most part, the more independent an adviser is from product-based compensation or compensation based on transaction volume, the better for the client. Costs do matter: keeping costs down is important, as is keeping advice independent of cost-inflating compensation methods. The crucial element, however, is the advisor's integrity— not the method of compensation.

The terms *fee-only* and *fee-based* are used as though they are interchangeable. They are different. In fact, you need to clarify the compensation method before you retain an adviser. (The most common method of compensation is still through commission fees.)

Fee-only means just that: the adviser is compensated *only* by fees paid by the client, with no commissions, trailers, finder's fees, or hidden remuneration paid to the adviser. Fee-only advisers are not licensed to sell any investment or life insurance products.

Fee-based means that the adviser may charge a fee to the client for services rendered, but that same adviser may also be entitled to a finder's fee, trailer fee, or other fee for having obtained the business or referred it on to an investment products provider.

Whatever type of investment advisor you choose, remember that it is your money (or that of your disabled relative or person for whom you are the legal representative). This means you should have the following expectations of your investment management firm:

- Above all, they put your interest first, not that of the advisor.
- They understand the overwhelming need for capital safety and an assured income flow.
- Investments are for the long term.
- They invest conservatively. This means investing at least 50% of the settlement in fixed income securities, but no more than 50% in high-quality equities, including some outside Canada.
- They invest in securities that you and your family understand. If you don't understand them, don't be talked into buying them.

Before selecting any kind of investment advisor, do your own research into what type of advisor you need! Read, ask questions, and understand the big picture in investing. You need to develop a written plan for investments and an overall financial plan. Once these plans have been developed, you must monitor them carefully.

Speaking from Experience...

Rose was hit by a car while riding her bike 20 years ago, at the age of 20. She was in a coma for several months and suffered a brain injury. A structured settlement was put in place that paid $300 per month for 10 years, $500 per month for 5 years, $1,500 per month at age 45 and, thereafter, adjusted for inflation each year. Although Rose has made a remarkable recovery and is now married with two wonderful *children, her career and working life have been severely limited as a result of the accident. The increases in the structured settlement ensure that, if she had needed long term care that could not be provided by her family, the increasing settlement payments would ensure she was taken care of in the future.*

Graham was in a bad car accident 20 years ago at the age of 34, which resulted in his becoming a quadriplegic. As a skilled tradesperson, he received a settlement of $950,000, out of which he had legal fees and other expenses that amounted to about $200,000. None of his settlement went into a structured settlement. Four years later, he and his wife divorced. As some of the settlement had been invested in rental real estate in his wife's name in order to minimize income taxes, she was entitled to claim a much larger portion of the family property than if some or all had gone into a structured settlement.

Lucille was paralyzed in a car accident when she was in her 20's. She was under the influence of her domineering father and her sister, and a "boy friend" who smelled money, each of whom made financial demands on her. The investment counsellors who managed the lump-sum settlement worked hard to make the money work for her so it would last as long as possible despite the depletions. One day, the firm that held the securities in trust was informed that the client wanted to move the funds to a stock brokerage account. The broker promised better returns than the "measly" 10% achieved by the investment counsellors in the market good times! Commented the investment counsellors, "One way or another, that settlement was being wasted away, and that client was going to be left on her own, a lonely, impoverished, and disabled woman."

SOURCES OF INFORMATION

Recommended Reading
(Due to recent upheavals in the Canadian publishing industry, many of the titles listed below may not be available for purchase. Check with your local bookstore or on-line, in the business and finance section. Also look in your local library.)

The Wealthy Barber, by David Chilton. This is the very basic book for those who need to learn how investment management "fits" in the larger world of financial planning.

The Money Adviser, by Bruce Cohen with Alyssa Diamond. This book gives an overview of financial and investment planning at a more detailed, but understandable, level.

The Insider's Guide to Selecting the Best Money Manager, by Kelly Rodgers. In this book, Ms. Rodgers discusses finding suitable investment counsellors for managing larger sums of money.

Investing for Dummies, by Eric Tyson and Tony Martin. John Wiley & Sons Canada. A book that concentrates on understanding investments and some of the players in the investment world in Canada.

Financial Pursuit, by Graydon G. Watters. A good overview of financial planning with illustrated sections on investing.

Risk is a Four Letter Word, and Risk is Still a Four Letter Word, by George Hartman. This gives the basics of risk/reward, asset allocation strategies. It is an easy-to-read primer.

Related Web Sites
The Canadian Securities Administrators, with links to provincial Securities Commissions across Canada: www.csa-acvm.ca Provincial listings give names of advisers, their companies and their licensing status.

The Investment Counsel Association of Canada. For information about finding investment counsellors: www.investmentcounsel.org

Advocis, the Financial Advisors Association of Canada. For information on selecting financial planners and advisors and insurance advisors: www.advocis.ca

Financial Planners Standards Council. For listings of members who hold the Certified Financial Planner (CFP) designation: www.cfp-ca.org

IAFP (Institute of Advanced Financial Planners) is the professional association for financial planners who hold the designation, Registered Financial Planner (RFP). www.iafp.ca

CIFP (Canadian Institute of Financial Planners) an association of Canadian financial planners. www.cifps.ca

Structured Settlements information supplied by McKellar Structured Settlements Inc. www.mckellar.com

CHAPTER 14

HOUSING ISSUES

After diagnosis, treatment and rehabilitation, the next question for a person with a disability is, "Where will I live?" For those with families the question is, "Where will *we* live?" Affordable, accessible housing for people with disabilities is in short supply all across Canada. Even if you own your home, the rules for assistance can be confusing and making the modifications can be costly.

AVAILABILITY OF ACCESSIBLE HOUSING

Slow onset disabilities such as multiple sclerosis, Parkinson's disease and similar conditions at least give people an opportunity to plan ahead for their accommodation. But people who are disabled suddenly, as with a spinal cord injury, brain injury, or stroke, likely have to deal with things in a hurry. In an informal cross-Canada survey of people with disabilities and those who work or live with them, everyone agreed that one of the biggest problems is the lack of accessible housing, whether it is affordable or not.

The health care system is focused on diagnosing and treating people and getting them home again (i.e., out of hospital) as quickly as possible. Ten years ago, most people with spinal cord injuries spent 2 years in rehabilitation. Today, it is rare for anyone to stay more than a year, and most people stay only 3 to 5 months, as did Janet (and former British Columbia premier Mike Harcourt.) People with disabilities requiring financial assistance must provide a great deal of information to the program reviewers—and the application can take months to process—leaving a person unable to go home and nowhere to live in the meantime. This also applies to those wanting rental housing.

What happens if no accessible housing is available in a community? Either the person with the disability remains in hospital for an extended period of time or, frequently, is moved into a long term care or seniors' residence. Living in a seniors' residence may not be a problem if the person with the disability is actually a senior, but there are many cases when young people, as young as 18 are placed in seniors' buildings. This is really not acceptable since young people face many psychological and social barriers in this setting, separated from other people in their own age group.

Janet's story

I reviewed the application forms for subsidized housing for me and my children during my rehabilitation. One of the things I noticed was that there are very few three-bedroom disabled apartments, and not very many more two-bedroom. It occurred to me that the message we get from this is that people with disabilities were not supposed to have families. The assumption was obviously being made that most of the people with disabilities were assumed to be young single men and women and old men and women. If I had to rely on social housing, and had not been able to move back into my own home or had not had the resources to enable me to be self-sufficient, I worry about where I would be now. The waiting list seems to be at least 5 years long. But in the meantime, where are the people supposed to go?

The federal government pulled out of subsidized housing in the early 1990s. Provinces have cut back drastically since then, too. Part of the problem is that some provinces have downloaded responsibility for social housing to municipalities. Recently, the federal government has promised to build more affordable housing. But housing remains a crisis for both able-bodied and disabled in many communities, particularly for people who require subsidized housing. In Toronto, the wait can easily be as long as 5 years or more for a housing subsidy. The other problem is that the needs of the homeless with disabilities are not necessarily addressed or understood.

There are essentially three sources of affordable, accessible housing in Canada: housing co-operatives, public housing, and housing sponsored by charitable organizations such as the Clarendon Foundation.

Housing Co-operatives

Canadians have been building and living in housing cooperatives since the 1930's, yet many people do not know about them or how they work. A housing co-op is a legal entity, a community, and a response to the need for decent, affordable housing.

As a legal entity, a housing co-op is a non-profit corporation, governed by provincial laws. If the co-op was developed with government funding, it will also have some kind of agreement with that level of government. People who live co-ops are *members* and they run the co-op through an elected board of directors. Members of a co-op "own" their homes collectively, though no members actually have equity. You cannot sell your home and realize the equity from it. The equity stays with the co-operative corporation if you move.

Co-ops tend to be less expensive to run than other kinds of housing, and that means the rents, or housing charges as they are called, *may* be lower than the regular rental market—though not necessarily. In addition, all housing co-ops can offer subsidies. About half of all co-op households pay a monthly charge geared to their income, usually about 30% of income. Government funds cover the difference between this payment and the co-op's costs. Because co-ops are run by members, the people who live in co-ops tend to have a greater say in how their buildings are run and maintained than in other forms of rental housing.

Today, there are about 2,100 non-profit housing co-ops across the country in every province and territory. They are home to about a quarter of a million people in 90,000 households. Over 5,000 co-operatively owned dwellings house one or more people with a physical disability. In fact, some jurisdictions *require* that all new co-ops have a number of already-modified units for people with disabilities. Housing co-ops also pride themselves on encouraging diversity among their members.

Housing co-ops could be a good alternative for people with disabilities, but there are often long waiting lists for membership in housing co-ops and even longer waiting lists for those needing subsidies.

Public Housing

There are long waiting lists for subsidized public housing units that are administered by municipalities. Some of these units are in high crime areas, which deter many people with disabilities from accepting these places since they now feel more vulnerable to criminals. Check with the rehabilitation counsellor at the rehabilitation facility in your community as well as the municipal housing office.

Charities

Many communities across Canada have set up housing facilities for people with disabilities through community initiatives or charitable organizations and foundations. Check with you local municipality for information. Also, contact various charities that sponsor housing projects across Canada.

How to apply

As mentioned above, getting into housing programs, whether co-ops or public housing or charity-sponsored housing, adds a layer of bureaucracy to the life of a person with a disability—when they least need it. Be prepared to fill out an application and provide verification of your income, your housing history, and a credit check for some of these programs. Co-ops may require an interview with a membership committee.

Home Modifications

For someone who owns his or her own home, there is the option of modifying it to suit the needs of the person with the disability. If at all possible, people considering this option should speak to others who have been through the process and learn from their mistakes and successes. (See "Sources of Information" at the end of this chapter.) There are also professionals who specialize in modifying homes for people with disabilities, but their advice comes at a price.

Generally, though, someone or several people from the rehabilitation centre—an occupational therapist, physiotherapist and/or discharge planner—will do an on-site inspection of your home before you are discharged. They will be looking for answers to two main questions:

- Can the person with the disability live in his or her present home as it is currently set up?
- Can the person live in the home if modifications are made to the home? If yes, what modifications must be made?

Modifications Required

The types of modification required will depend very much on the nature of the disability. For example, the modifications required for a person using a wheelchair for mobility will be different from those needed for a person with a visual impairment, or for a person with Alzheimer's. The following are some typical modifications:

- Installation of ramps or special railings to access the home

- Installation of elevators or stair-glides so that the person can move from one floor to the next
- Reconfiguring bathrooms, including new flooring, grab-bars, removal of carpeting, installing a large, barrier-free shower, special tubs, equipping the bathroom with a bath chair and hand-held shower
- Widening doorways
- Adjusting counter and cupboard heights in kitchens
- Electrical outlets placed at convenient height for people in wheelchairs
- Replacing uneven or carpeted flooring with hardwood or tile
- Equipping the kitchen with safe electrical appliances, such as automatic shut-off kettles
- Replacing door knobs or twist sink taps with lever-style controls

Canada Mortgage and Housing Corporation (CMHC) has a checklist for home modifications. (See "Sources of Information" at the end of this chapter).

FEDERAL FUNDING PROGRAMS

Canada Mortgage and Housing Corporation Residential Rehabilitation Assistance Program for Persons with Disabilities

The Canada Mortgage and Housing Corporation (CMHC) is a federal government agency that administers the Residential Rehabilitation Assistance Program for Persons with Disabilities program (RRAP-D). The RRAP-D program offers financial assistance to homeowners with disabilities and to landlords to make modifications to residences to make them accessible to lower income people with disabilities. In some provinces, the program is delivered through the provincial or territorial housing agency.

The RRAP-D assistance is structured as a loan, some or all of which may be forgiven over a period of time. The amounts available vary from location to location across the country. (See chart.)

For landlords, CMHC may forgive 100% of the loan for accessibility modifications so long as the units continue to be affordable and new occupancy is limited to households with incomes below the threshold for that area.

For homeowners, the forgivable amount varies according to household income and the cost of the accessibility modifications. A repayable loan may be given above the forgivable portion up to the maximum loan available. To be eligible for forgiveness, the homeowner must agree to own and occupy the home for 5 years, and then the loan is forgiven by a portion each year. Maximum forgiveness is available when the household income is 60% or less of the income threshold for the area and family size. (See chart.)

The CMHC Web site lists current maximum amounts:

	Maximum Loan (Homeowner/Landlord)	Maximum Forgiveness (Homeowner)
Zone 1: Southern areas Of Canada	$18,000	$12,000
Zone 2: Northern Areas	$21,000	$14,000
Zone 3: Far Northern Areas	$27,000	$18,000

Who qualifies?

The definition of disability under the plan is "any person who, because of one or more persistent physical, psychiatric, learning, or sensory disabilities, is unable to ensure himself/herself the necessities or social life of a person without a disability." After a serious disability, as a result of which the person is unable to work and the family has limited means, it is likely that the person will qualify for this program.

For homeowners, CMHC considers family income and the value of the home when assessing the application. The applicant does not have to be in receipt of social assistance to be considered. The location of the property is also considered. There is a cap based on the assessed value of the home. Homeowners with properties valued higher than the cap will not get assistance. For example, in Toronto in 2003, the amount is $250,000 of assessed value, which is likely below market value.

Landlords whose property meets minimum health and safety standards (including rooming houses) can apply for grants if their units are at or below established value levels and if the units are occupied by tenants whose income levels are within CMHC's guidelines for maximum income.

What modifications qualify?

Although people assume that the modifications are essentially for people who use wheelchairs, the program is much broader than that. It can be also be used for improvements to the property that enable partially sighted people to be better able to function in their home environment or to install a security system in cases where a member of the family may have a tendency to wander. It is very common for people applying for RRAP-D to ask for air conditioning, but only in very rare cases is this an allowable improvement.

Modifications that qualify for RRAP-D must be related to housing and be reasonably related to the person's disability. Many proposed structural improvements qualify under this program. Most modifications that allow a person to live independently will qualify, such as a ramp, chair lift, bathtub lift, wheel-in shower, suitable height adjustments to kitchen workspace and cupboards, and handrails. Stair-glides are eligible as they are considered structural improvements because they are bolted to the staircase and connected into the electricity supply.

Therapeutic items such as mobility devices (wheelchairs and walkers) and most household appliances are *not* eligible.

Loans for accessibility modifications are given only if they have been approved in advance of renovations being made. In short, CMHC will not reimburse you for accessibility renovations already completed. The approval time can take anywhere from a month—if all the information is submitted with the application—to a year or more if the information is incomplete.

General RRAP Program

CMHC also administers a RRAP program for low-income homeowners to upgrade their homes to bring them up to standard in the areas of plumbing, heating, electrical, structural, or fire safety. Homeowners may qualify under both RRAP and RRAP-D programs.

Some points to remember:
- The qualifying loan depends upon how many family members there are and how many income earners there are.
- Those who can potentially benefit from this program should get information early on in their disability so that they can apply as soon as possible.
- The income level cut-off is not very high, given that persons with disabilities have other financial burdens (such as additional health care costs, home help, etc.) However, it is significantly higher than provincial welfare income cut-offs.
- Persons with disabilities who are recipients of workers' compensation housing modification benefits are not eligible for RRAP programs.

Ontario March of Dimes Home and Vehicle Modification Program

Few other provinces have programs that compare with the Ontario March of Dimes Home and Vehicle Modification Program. It has been in operation for several years and is run by the Ontario March of Dimes with funding from the Ontario Ministry of Community, Family, and Children's Services. The program provides funding of up to $15,000 to residents of Ontario over the age of 18 toward the cost of home and/or vehicle modifications. They serve about 308 clients through an annual budget of $2.2 million. The average grant, therefore, is about $7,000.

The program's aims are as follows:

- Prevent hospitalization or institutionalization
- Eliminate risks to personal safety
- Permit earlier discharge from institutions
- Avoid loss of employment or income

Who qualifies?

The program is designed for adults with disabilities expected to last at least 1 year. There is a family income cut-off of $65,000. Above that income, no grant will be paid. Families with incomes of $35,000 to $65,000, may have to contribute toward the cost of the modifications.

Homes must be owned by the applicant or a close family member. Be aware, however, that if the house is owned by a family member, the family member's income will be used in calculations determining eligibility.

Applicants living in rented units may be eligible to receive transferable installed equipment such as ceiling track lifts, automated door openers, etc. Landlords of tenants with a disability are not eligible for funding through this program (but likely would be through RRAP-D).

Applicants must exhaust all other sources of funding before applying. This means that if the applicant has a claim under any other insurance, or there is a settlement that is expected quite soon, those sources of funding have to be used first. The program also works in conjunction with the RRAP-D program when appropriate and funding may be split between the two programs.

There is no typical recipient of these funds. Recipients include young people disabled as children who are leaving home; people in mid-career; people disabled as a result of accident, injury, or disease.

What qualifies?

Applicants may be eligible for $15,000 for home modifications and $15,000 for vehicle modifications. When there are two or more people with disabilities in a household, the maximum applies per household not per individual. Applicants moving from accessible to inaccessible housing are not eligible for funding.

Most grants are for home modifications. There are a number of restrictions and requirements, listed below. Work must *not* begin until approval has been granted or payment will not be made.

Restrictions:

- The funds may not be used to purchase a new vehicle or home. They may be used only for modifications to the current home or vehicle.
- Home modifications are available one time only. Vehicle modifications may be given once every 10 years.
- Vendors and contractors must not be related to the applicant.
- Vehicle modifications will not be given if there is a safe accessible, transit system. (Therefore, vehicle modifications are not normally granted in large metropolitan areas where accessible transit is available.)
- Modifications to newly constructed homes cannot be funded through this program.

- Vehicle modification grants are only given for vehicles owned by applicants or immediate family members. Leased or rented vehicles are not eligible.
- The minimum amount for any modification is $500.

How to apply

There are three periods when people can apply to the Ontario March of Dimes program: January 1 to February 15, May 1 to June 15, and September 1 to October 15. Applications will not be considered for funding if they are submitted outside these periods. Annual funding is apportioned equally for the three application periods. Those applicants with the most critical needs will be given priority. If an applicant does not receive funding, they can reapply for the next period. Applicants are notified within 90 days of the opening of the application window whether they have been successful or not.

At the beginning of this program, there was a huge backlog and many people had to be denied funding. The backlog seems to have been resolved, and there is nothing to prevent people from reapplying for funding under the new rules (assuming work has not started.)

The application form

The application form requires a lot of detailed information and a lot of documentation. It includes a self-screening tool to prevent applicants from claiming items that are not covered under the program. If the total cost of the project (home or vehicle) is above the maximum, you must provide documentation that you can quickly get access to additional funds. Other information and documentation required:

Homes

- An occupational therapist's report linking modifications to the consumer's needs

- Two quotes from qualified contractors/vendors based on the occupational therapist's assessment
- Documentation that the home is in good condition and meets fire safety standards and other local building codes and will still do so after the modifications. This includes photographs of all areas to be modified plus the front façade of the property.

Vehicles
- Documentation that the principal driver has a valid driver's licence
- Proof that the vehicle is owned by the applicant or family member and is safe to drive
- Evidence that the owner can afford to maintain and insure the vehicle.

Appeals
Decisions based on lack of available funding cannot be appealed. Decisions that deny funding approval for specific items also cannot be appealed. Applicants who have initially been denied funding on the basis of their eligibility may appeal, however.

Other provinces
Although none of the other provinces have such wide-reaching programs, Alberta has a program known as the Home Adaptation Program. Under this program, if a family's gross annual income is under $25,000, they qualify for up to $5,000 for home modifications providing there is a family member who uses (or will soon use) a wheelchair. If family income is between $25,000 and $32,000, the grant is $2,500. Above income of $32,000 there is no grant available.

Without this type of program in place, residents of other provinces will have to approach charities and service clubs.

CMHC Flexhouse

Although CMHC Flexhouse funding is not a source for modifications, it is a new approach to housing design developed in 1995. The idea is to design and build housing that is easily adaptable in the long term for people with disabilities. With an aging population that is going to require more accessible housing, planning ahead will save money.

The Flexhouse designs adapt to changes in a family's lifestyle without forcing them to move—rooms can change in size and function; living spaces are accessible and functional to meet a family's needs, whatever they are.

Flexhouse designs show the principles of universal, barrier-free design in practice. For example, electrical outlets are installed at a suitable height for people in wheelchairs; driveways are wider to enable a wheelchair user to access a vehicle; bathrooms allow turning space for a wheelchair.

Retro-fitting a home is expensive: smart home builders and home buyers are asking for adaptable, barrier-free home and apartment designs at the outset of a project. All consumers appreciate wider doorways and adaptable kitchens.

You can get Flex housing details from CMHC (Pocket Planner, Homes that Adapt).

Why Good Design for People with Disabilities Matters

Speaking from Experience...

Wheelchair washrooms—the people who design them have no idea about people who need to do intermittent catheterization. In most washrooms there is nowhere to put the supplies and swabs and so on. And half the time, you couldn't possibly get a wheelchair next to the toilet to transfer. At the Shaw festival they have a lovely huge disabled washroom but the lighting is so bad, that I couldn't see what I was doing! Lovely mood lighting! We need a garbage can with a lid that stays up and a little table to put supplies on. And enough light to see what you are doing. Some of them you can't turn a wheelchair around in. We also need a washbasin in the washroom [toilet enclosure] to help with hygiene. The door needs to be automatic too or not too heavy to push.

The same applies to some workplaces. At the hospital where I worked, there wasn't a button to get in to the washroom and the door was too heavy to manoeuvre in a wheelchair. The reasoning was that since the washroom was for patients and it was a children's hospital, the kids would have someone with them!

Community Living

There are several organizations in each province that operate sheltered housing or community living environments. These assisted housing facilities are for individuals who require close supervision or assistance from attendants because of the nature of their disabilities.

People with severe brain injuries are placed in such facilities when space is available. For example, 19% of adults with brain injury live alone; 58% are cared for by families. Only 5% live in community residences and 9% in institutions. By contrast, among children with brain injuries, 88% are cared for by families and 9% live in institutions.

In short, community living options are very limited and there are never enough spaces available. In many cases, community living spaces are not available (because of shortage of supply) until the caregivers are in their eighties and the person with a disability is well into middle age.

Speaking from Experience...

Tom's comments:

On the issue of building larger group residences to be occupied by people with disabilities, none of us want to see that happen in Canada. It sets us back and marginalizes people with disabilities. And really that's all we are—people who happen to have a physical disability. We shouldn't be segregated from the Main Street population, because passing somebody in a wheelchair today, you could be in the same bloody situation tomorrow!

There are significant differences between rural and urban communities. Smaller communities are much more likely to rally round and fundraise for residents with disabilities who need equipment and have other needs that are not being met by government funding. There are also examples of local communities setting up sheltered housing and community living communities.

SOURCES OF INFORMATION

Canadian Association of Community Living Organizations www.cailc.ca
There are links to community living sites across Canada, province-by-province at this site.
Canadian Federation of Housing Co-ops www.cfhc.coop
Use this site to access the Web sites for provincial housing co-operatives federations. From the provincial sites, you will be able to get to the sites of individual co-ops.
www.scipilot.com *SCIPILOT* stands for Spinal Cord Injury Peer Information Library on Technology. A project of the Lyndhurst Spinal Cord Centre in Toronto, it contains over 40 first–person stories obtaining and using assistive technology. Most stories include hints and tips for people adapting housing to their needs.

CMHC guides:

Housing for persons with disabilities NHA 5467 provides diagrams and explanations of basic design features and dimensions to improve accessibility.

How to hire a Contractor — a guide to selecting a contractor, obtaining bids and estimates, supervising the work and getting satisfactory results.

A Modification Checklist — accessibility using RRAP for persons with disabilities

CMHC Web site www.cmhc-schl.gc.ca

Ontario March of Dimes:

Home & Vehicle Modification Program
700 Richmond St, Suite 310
London, Ont. N6A 5C7
Tel: 1877-369-4867
TTY: 519-642-3999
Web site: www.dimes.on.ca

Useful publications:

Where Will They Live? A Guide to Help You Help Your Parents with Their Housing Decisions, by Barbara H. Carter. Stoddart, 2002. Primarily intended for adult children helping senior parents, this is also a useful resource for those assisting disabled adults of any age.

Solutions, Canada's Family Guide to Home Health Care and Wellness magazine, published quarterly by BCS Communications Ltd., 101 Thorncliffe Park Drive, Toronto, ON M4H 1M2 www.bcsgroup.com Also by the same publisher, Rehab & Community Care Management.

CHAPTER 15

ATTENDANT CARE SERVICES AND EQUIPMENT FUNDING

There are two types of attendant care services available in most provinces. The first is *attendant care* and the second is *self-managed attendant care.*

ATTENDANT CARE

What Is Attendant Care?

When people with disabilities are discharged from rehabilitation, they may need help with some of the functions of daily living. Some of the additional services needed may be met by home care (see Chapter 16, "Miscellany: After Care, Home Care, Caregiving Issues"), or paid for through extended health benefits (see Chapter 5, "Employee Benefit and Individual Plans"). But the level of services required by some people is significantly higher than that provided through these systems. This is where *attendant care* comes in.

Attendant care includes non-medical services that are directed by the person with a disability who requires assistance with such activities as:

- Personal grooming and hygiene
- Bathing, toileting, and bowel routine
- Transferring to and from bed
- Dressing and undressing
- Light housekeeping and meal preparation
- Assistance with medications

Attendant care services do not include physiotherapy, rehabilitation, life skills teaching, active nursing, socializing, etc. In Ontario, these services are provided through Community Care Access Centres (Home Care), and by equivalent agencies in other provinces.

Who qualifies for attendant care?

In most provinces, those who normally qualify are those people who are unable to get out of bed or into bed on their own and those who need a considerable amount of help with the activities of daily living other than what can be provided by home care services.

In addition, the person with the physical disability must:

- Be at least 16 years old
- Have a permanent physical disability and require assistance with the activities of daily living
- Be able to direct their own care
- Have attendant services provided in their own home
- Have the attendant care service provided in their workplace or educational facility, when appropriate

Who pays for Attendant Care?

In Ontario (and most other provinces), attendant care is fully funded by the Ministry of Health, but service delivery can be through a variety of different agencies. For example, in Ontario both the Canadian Paraplegic Association Ontario and the Ontario March of Dimes provide attendant services for adults who have physical disabilities and wish to direct their own care while living at home. This also allows people with disabilities to be employed. In fact, having attendant care may mean the difference between working and unemployment.

Remember, attendant care does not replace home care, but rather is in addition to what home care might provide. Home care is not available as a 24-hour a day service, nor is it available on an on-call or emergency basis. But attendant care is often provided as a 24-hour service or on an emergency basis.

SELF-MANAGED ATTENDANT SERVICES: DIRECT FUNDING

What is Self-Managed Attendant Care?

From the patient's perspective, one of the problems with attendant care is having control over the care provided and ensuring the best care for themselves. Many people with disabilities who use wheelchairs suggested, and lobbied for, changes to the attendant care funding system that allows them to hire their own attendants.

The issue of letting people with disabilities regain as much control over their lives as possible is extremely important. Nowhere is it more so than in the opportunity to not only direct their own care, but also to choose who is going to administer that care. The person with the disability becomes the employer of the attendant and is fully responsible for managing a budget and accounting for the expenditure of funds granted by the provincial government. Normally, this budget includes an amount to pay for bookkeeping.

The direct funding option offers several advantages. It allows the person with a disability:

- To be in charge of their own staffing and scheduling of the attendant to meet *their* needs.
- To selectively hire people based on the disabled person's individual requirements. Therefore, if there is a language issue, an attendant can be hired who speaks the same language as the person with the disability. Gender of the attendant can also be an issue—generally speaking, people with disabilities prefer an attendant of the same sex.
- To live anywhere in the province

Direct funding is an option suited to people with physical disabilities who are able and willing to take on the extra management responsibilities that the program demands.

Who Qualifies for Direct Funding?

The following criteria must be met in order to qualify for direct funding under the Direct Funding Program administered by the Centre for Independent Living in Toronto (CILT) as outlined in their Web site description of the program (www.cilt.ca). These criteria are typical of direct funding programs in other provinces which offer such programs.

- The person with the disability must be able to self-direct, which means that you know your disability and needs and can instruct your attendants as to how and when you need assistance. You must be able to help train the attendants accordingly.
- In addition, you must be able to *self-manage*. The self-manager is a person in control of his or her own situation and not easily manipulated. A self-manager is a person who knows what services he or she wants and needs, someone with plans—perhaps to move, work or study—or simply a clear desire to take responsibility for improving his or her own services. You must be willing to take risks in return for the choice, flexibility, and control over your attendant services made possible under direct funding.

In addition, in order to qualify in Ontario you must be a resident, aged 16 or over, require attendant services due to a permanent physical disability and the following more specific requirements as outlined in the program as described on the CILT Web site, you must be able to:

- Complete the written application on your own initiative and in your own words, although you may receive physical assistance to complete the form. However, submissions may not be made by professionals, family members or others on your behalf
- Meet with a selection panel to discuss your needs and determine your eligibility for the program

- Schedule attendants
- Hire (and fire if necessary), train and supervise one or more attendant workers
- Meet all the legal requirements associated with being an employer
- Manage and account for your funding according to direct-funding guidelines.

Note that the responsibilities of an employer as outlined above cannot be assumed by any other person on behalf of the person with the disability. Management by family members or power of attorney is not permitted under direct funding guidelines.

What does Self-Managed Attendant Care Cover?

People have different needs so the level of service required by each person will vary. In Ontario, the funding provides for no more than an average of 6 hours per day or 182.5 hours per month. However, people who need assistance with breathing may be eligible for more funded hours of assistance.

What are the benefits of Self-Managed Attendant Care?

There are other benefits to direct funding in addition to controlling your own care. For example, there is greater flexibility allowed in arranging for attendant services, which are paid at the regular hourly wage rate, plus a flat rate, which can also be paid for indirect services. For instance, you could arrange for an attendant to stay overnight, or to carry a pager for emergency assistance, or to offer an attendant room and board as a means of extending coverage over more hours in the day.

Employer Responsibilities

Not only must the person with the disability who is employing an attendant be able to manage money, time,

and personnel, they must also be able to do the
following:

- Apply for a business number from Canada
  Customs and Revenue Agency;
- Make payroll deductions related to the Canada
  Pension Plan, Employment Insurance, income tax,
  and workers compensation
- Comply with provincial labour standards and
  human rights legislation
- Follow occupational health and safety standards
  and workplace safety and insurance requirements

Once screening has been completed and a participant
is accepted into the program, there is a legally binding
agreement drawn up between the participant and the
program manager. This specifies allowable expenditures
and is monitored closely. If there is a misuse of funds or
any breach of the agreement, the participant may be
subject to legal action and no longer be allowed to
participate in the program. If participants need to
change their care, the program can be adjusted to
reflect this and a participant may voluntarily withdraw
from the program at any time.

However, in the case of people living in supportive
housing where attendant care services are provided on-
site, once they are accepted into the direct funding
program, they have to move out of the supportive
housing unit within 3 months in order to continue to
receive direct funding.

There are other program conditions:

- Participants may not hire or pay immediate family
  members—including parents, children, siblings,
  spouses or the equivalent—to provide services,
  including bookkeeping.
- Participants are responsible for training their own
  attendants. However, if special training is required
  there may be training available within the
  community free of charge. The local resource
  centre will have further information on this.

- Funds may be used anywhere within the province but not in a different province. If you move to another province you would have to apply in the new province for funding. However, you can move anywhere within the province and funding will not be affected.

Other Provinces

Most other provinces have similar programs in place allowing disabled people to direct their own care. At time of writing, Saskatchewan does not yet have a program in place. Several Maritime provinces have pilot projects in place. In Ontario, the program currently provides funding for 700 people living with disabilities.

At present, the Ontario program is full and there is a waiting list for applications. This is a problem for people who want the ability to have more control over their lives. Since the program is designed for people who are able to work or go to school, the chances are this form of funding for them will continue long term. Therefore, new applicants may have a very long wait to obtain this type of funding unless the program is expanded to meet current and future needs.

EQUIPMENT FUNDING

Depending on the type of disability, people may need various pieces of equipment to help them maintain as much functional independence as possible, as well as ensuring their safety. The costs of equipment can be extremely expensive. For someone whose income may already be dramatically reduced, it may be prohibitive. People whose disability arises from an injury or disease where they can sue or receive other forms of compensation (such as worker's compensation or a motor vehicle accident claim) will have all their equipment needs met by that program, or it will form part of the settlement.

But there are a large number of people with disabilities who fall through the cracks. There are, however, some programs designed to help with this.

Firstly, most provinces run some sort of *Assistive Devices* program (ADP). In most of the provinces, this program is *only* available to those on social assistance. In Ontario, the program is more universal in nature. The following is taken from the Ontario Assistive Devices Program Web site.

Objectives

The Assistive Devices Program (ADP) is administered by the Operational Support Branch of the Ontario Ministry of Health and Long Term Care.

The objective of ADP is to financially assist Ontario residents with long term physical disabilities to obtain basic, competitively priced, personalized assistive devices appropriate for the individual's needs and essential for independent living.

Devices covered by the program are intended to give people increased independence and control over their lives. They may allow people to avoid costly institutional settings and remain in the community.

Equipment Funded by ADP

Ontario ADP covers over 8,000 separate pieces of equipment or supplies in the following categories:
- Prostheses
- Wheelchairs/mobility aids and specialized seating systems
- Ostomy, and enteral feeding supplies
- Needles and syringes for insulin-dependent seniors
- Monitors and test stripes for insulin-dependent diabetics (through agreement with the Canadian Diabetes Association)
- Hearing aids
- Respiratory equipment

- Orthoses (braces, garments and pumps)
- Visual and communication aids
- Oxygen and oxygen delivery equipment, such as concentrators, cylinders, liquid systems and related supplies, such as masks and tubing.

Eligibility

Any Ontario resident who has a valid Ontario Health card issued in their name and has a physical disability of 6 months or longer is eligible to apply.

Equipment cannot be required exclusively for sports, work, or school but must be needed for normal daily activities.

There are specific eligibility criteria that apply to each device category.

Residents with a primary diagnosis of a learning or mental disability are excluded from ADP, as are those on workers' compensation.

Accessing ADP

Initial access is often through a medical specialist or general practitioner who provides a diagnosis. In most device categories, an *authorizer* assesses the specific needs of the person and prescribes appropriate equipment or supplies. Finally, a *vendor* sells the equipment or supplies to the client.

In some device categories, such as adult hearing aids or prosthetic devices, the assessor is also the vendor (seller).

Authorizer

Most devices must be authorized by a qualified health care professional registered with the program. Registered authorizers work in hospitals, home care agencies or in private practice.

Vendor

The program will help pay only for equipment that is purchased from vendors registered with the Assistive Devices Program.

Financial Assistance

ADP pays up to 75% of the cost of equipment, such as artificial limbs, orthopaedic braces, wheelchairs, breast prostheses, and breathing aids. For others, such as hearing aids, the ADP contributes a fixed amount. With regard to supply items as ostomy and needles and syringes for seniors, the ADP pays an annual grant directly to the person. The home oxygen program, under ADP, pays 100% of the cost of. oxygen and related equipment for seniors and those on social assistance, home care, or residing in a long term care facility, and 75% for all others.

In most cases, the client pays a share of the cost at time of purchase and the vendor bills ADP the balance.

For ADP supply categories where grants are paid, the client pays 100% of the cost to the vendor.

All ages are eligible for devices, except the needles and syringes grant, which is restricted to insulin dependent seniors.

There are many sources of funding for the client's share of the cost including:

- Clients
- Voluntary/charitable organizations e.g. March of Dimes, Easter Seals, Kiwanis
- Social assistance,
- Department of Veterans Affairs
- Insurance companies
- Relatives/friends.

Commentary:

According to correspondents surveyed across Canada, it appears that in most provinces, an assistive devices program (ADP) is available only for people who are in receipt of social assistance payments.

Although accessing the ADP sounds very simple and straightforward, it is actually quite complex.

For example, wheelchair needs are divided into categories and, depending upon the level of injury, the person with the disability will fit into a certain category. It may be that a person may not qualify for a wheelchair, but rather will need a walker. Within the categories, there are specific wheelchairs at varying costs and, depending on the one chosen by the authorizer, the government will fund according to their notion of what the cost is. The Ontario government has not raised their prices in about 5 years, but of course the vendors have raised their prices over that period of time. So, in effect, the province is not paying 75%. Occasionally it happens that the province does pay 75%, if you have a low-end or inexpensive wheelchair in your category. (This is not always a smart move if you have to spend 12 to 15 hours per day in the wheelchair.) If the wheelchair has more accessories or more flexibility, or is made of lightweight material, it is less likely to be covered. Nor will those with more expensive backs or more expensive seats be covered. In these cases, the only hope is that an insurance plan may pick up the cost.

Other mobility devices that are covered include walkers, but items such as stair glides are not covered. Additional items such as a frame to hold a book, a mirror (to see behind when outside) and so on are not covered and the costs are high—a small plastic support for a cane costs $40! It may be that the assistive devices program serves to make the costs higher since there is the perception that the government in Ontario is paying 75% anyway.

Ontario theoretically picks up the additional 25% of the cost not covered by ADP for people on social assistance, but since they are often working with out of date pricing, in effect they are not really picking up the whole balance in many cases. This is because of the same problem outlined above, where ADP is basing the amount it pays on 5-year-old pricing.

Rehabilitation consultants say that it is quite common to see funding for a manual wheelchair when the client really requires an electric wheelchair. And, in many cases the client requires both. Clients then have to come up with the money themselves or contact a charitable foundation. There are not many charitable foundations providing funding for this type of expense. Mostly, there are grants of $300 to $500 when the need may be for $2,000 to $5,000.

For detailed insights into people's experiences dealing with decisions and purchases of wheelchairs and other assistive technology, you can read the stories of people with spinal cord injuries at www.scipilot.com.

Welfare uses the same pricing model as ADP, which causes the same problems. So in many cases when buying assistive technology, there is still an outstanding amount, which must be paid by the person with the disability.

Again, the person must look for money through charitable foundations and service organizations to help with funding. Easter Seals for youngsters and March of Dimes can be a major funder in this area in Ontario. Local service clubs are also an important resource. As helpful as these service clubs are, there needs to be more generous funding in this area by provincial governments. A manual wheelchair averages $3,000 and an electric wheelchair is $8-10,000 which can easily escalate, depending on the type of back, seat, head controls and tilting mechanisms, to $25,000 or even 45,000, if it is a wheelchair that allows a person to stand. That's the price of an SUV!

Computer Equipment

As a result of some types of disability, a person may not be able to communicate in all normal ways. Loss of the ability to speak, write or see can severely hamper a person's ability to get on with their life. A computer can assist enormously by using technology such as voice recognition software.

Some government funding is available for these programs, but it varies from province to province.

In other cases, disability insurance may provide benefits if the person with a disability needs resources to enable them to return to work.

Speaking from Experience...

Janet's story

My disability insurance company paid for voice recognition software (and training) to enable me to write financial planning reports. Although I have use of both hands, the fingers on my right hand cannot type well and I often have to type long reports (as well as this book!) The voice recognition software enabled me to work again.

Victor's story

After 8 months of waiting, Janet's neighbour, Victor, finally got a new wheelchair about 18 months ago through welfare. But it is already breaking down. He has to be in it for at least 8 hours per day. He is not overly hard on it and takes care of it, yet because it was a cheaply made model, it will not last.

Dave's story

Dave has spina bifida and is now in his forties. One of his ongoing problems has been bedsores, which has *resulted in many months of hospitalization and rehabilitation. His doctor and therapists have recommended a tilting wheelchair but ADP won't pay for it. His mother has had to pay $1,000 out of her own pocket.*

Janet's story

I had to buy my stair glide—I bought a used one which cost $2,400 installed. Neither ADP nor my extended health plan would pay anything towards it. (I didn't know that I could have received funding through the Residential Rehabilitation Assistance Program, discussed in Chapter 14.) When I tried to resell it 18 months later, I was told it was too old, and since the prices of new ones had come down I was offered $300! I have donated it to a charity and received a $500 donation receipt for it!

Extended Health Coverage for Assistive Devices

Some extended health insurance companies will fund the portion of the equipment, especially wheelchairs and other mobility devices, not covered by provincial programs. But often there are very specific requirements for what they will and won't cover as well as a dollar cap. For example, a stair glide is not covered by any of the extended health plans as it is considered to be a structural improvement to the home and not a mobility device, because of the fact that there is a frame that is attached to the staircase. Since the costs for new stair glides can be from $3,000 to $6,000 or more, buying one is a serious cash outlay.

Municipal programs

Even in Ontario, not all equipment is funded by the ADP program. Some items, such as bath benches, may not be covered, but some municipalities have assistance programs through social services. The problem here is that the funding available depends on the wealth of the municipality and the size of the tax base. For example, residents in Toronto may be entitled to more assistance than residents of Thunder Bay.

Charitable programs

The March of Dimes does a lot of fundraising for assistive devices (mainly mobility devices) through its own fundraising campaigns and in association with other charities and service clubs. Easter Seals, the sister organization of March of Dimes, which operates in most provinces, provides support and funding to children, but not to adults. Organizations working with people with specific diseases and disabilities may also assist with fundraising for mobility devices.

However, as noted above, some items such as stair glides are not considered mobility devices but rather home modifications or capital improvements. Funding for home modification or capital improvements is available through other programs such as CMHC Residential Rehabilitation Assistance Program for Persons with Disabilities (RRAP-D) plus the general RRAP program. (See Chapter 14, "Housing Issues.")

Rental programs

Several charities offer rental programs for equipment that may be required in the shorter term. In addition, most charities working with people with disabilities will accept donations of equipment that is no longer needed as long as it is in good working order, since most do not have the budget to repair equipment other than very minor repairs.

The Red Cross has an equipment loan or rental program in New Brunswick, Nova Scotia, and Prince Edward Island. Information is available on the Red Cross Web site.

Sometimes, it is possible to purchase used equipment, but especially with items such as stair glides and wheelchairs, what is suitable for one person does not necessarily meet the requirements of another. In other words, most items need to be custom fitted.

Some charities, such as the Multiple Sclerosis Society also loan, rather than rent, equipment to people with MS who cannot afford to purchase equipment themselves. Again, donations are readily accepted, and a charitable receipt will be issued for the depreciated value of the gift.

SOURCES OF INFORMATION

Ontario:
Assistive Devices Program
5700 Yonge Street, 7th Floor
Toronto, Ontario M2M 4K5
Or call:
Toronto: 416-327-8804
Toll Free: 1-800-268-6021
TDD/TTY: 416-327-4282
Toll Free: 1-800-387-5559
Web site: www.gov.on.ca
Canadian Association of Independent Living Centres www.cailc.ca
Canadian Red Cross Society www.redcross.ca
Spinal Cord Injured Peer Technology Information Library on Technology, www.scipilot.com. This site has firsthand accounts and advice from wheelchair users on equipment funding and related issues.

See Resource section at the back of the book for a listing of charities and other provincial government Web sites.

CHAPTER 16

MISCELLANY: AFTER CARE, HOME CARE, CAREGIVING ISSUES

Treatment or Rehabilitation; Short Term or Long Term

As discussed by Dr. Murray Waldman in Chapter 1, the medicare system in Canada focuses on diagnosis and treatment. This means that it is designed to find the problem and fix it. Thus, a person diagnosed with cancer is given treatment appropriate to that cancer (radiation, chemotherapy, etc.); a broken neck is diagnosed, surgery and treatment follows. But once the treatment is given, that is where medicare stops.

Janet's story

What this meant was that, while in my case I could walk, I needed ongoing physiotherapy beyond that for which the medical system was prepared to pay. Once I could walk a certain distance in a certain time frame— that was it. But after 6 months with no physiotherapy, I realized that I needed more treatment. The cost was $75 for a 45 minute session. If I had needed (or wanted) treatment at home, it would have been a lot more. In my case, I could afford to pay and also had made significant improvement such that I was able to look after myself and get around. But many people need ongoing intensive physiotherapy and occupational therapy to maintain the function they had by the time they left the hospital setting. And much of that therapy needs to be delivered in the home. My extended health care insurance pays $40 per session for just six sessions per year.

From the care provider's perspective, Dr. Murray Waldman observes:

Rehabilitation doesn't fit the medicare model—diagnosis and treatment—and so it always gets short shrift from medicare funding programs. And it's going to become more of an issue. This issue of getting better and feeling better is terribly, terribly important when you talk of an ageing population. Because we all have stuff that we are not going to get better from—but we want to feel better. So we want to be able to still function. The choice is really either to remove rehabilitation from the medical model or change the medical model to encompass rehabilitation. The chances of changing the model in Canada are almost zero because the implications for costs are huge. If you say that people will have the right to rehab and to get back to the function they had before, without reference to how they became dysfunctional, it opens up the door to huge amounts of costs. Most people as they get older could use some form of aid, whether it's mechanical or human. So this is always the big problem, to get people to accept disability as an issue.

The Romanow Commission on Health Care final report makes recommendations to include rehabilitation under the Canada Health Act for patients after they have received acute care. This would be a good start, but this is still short-term rehabilitation. There have been many stories in the newspapers of people well into their eighties trying to care for spouses and adult children or grandchildren. Home care has been cut, even as demand increases. The trend over the past 15 years has been to dramatically cut hospital stays without ploughing some of the savings back into home care.

Home Care

Janet's story

Home care was set up before I left the hospital—5 days a week, 2 hours per day. I needed help with bathing, meal preparation, and laundry as well as occasional shopping, which friends did for me.

I was supposed to be getting a caregiver every day as well as home physiotherapy and occupational therapy. The caregiver (called a Personal Support Worker to "give them more respect!") came on Monday; Tuesday she phoned at 3 p.m. to tell me she'd be here after 4. I sat in the living room waiting for her and she never came. The story on Wednesday morning was that she came and I wasn't here! The door was left unlocked for her and the back door, too, so I don't think she came. I know it is difficult to get good people. What bothered me was that it wasn't monitored if she did or did not come—I could have been lying on the floor in a pool of blood and nobody would have acted on it!

The "Personal Services Worker" provided by my local Community Care Access Centre was fine. I had no problems with her. But I don't think I ever got 2 hours per day. It was impossible for her. She typically had eight patients a day and was supposed to spend at least 2 hours with each. That's 16 hours or more per day. She had young children at home, too.

The first visit I had from someone from Home Care was about 2 weeks after I came home. They were doing an assessment. She didn't think I should have home care and told me that I would not be eligible for 5 days per week for long—and that I only needed a bath once per week. I don't have serious incontinence problems, but I have some.

Soon after, I was cut back to 3 times per week and then to twice per week. Around this time—after 3 months—I had a visit from the supervisor. When she arrived my homemaker answered the door—in her uniform and all—and the supervisor thought she was me! Even my worker thought she was dumb! At the end of January, my worker came in one day and said this is my last visit. So I was very upset and called the supervisor. She hadn't called back after three messages so I called the manager, and then she called me. She accused me of malingering and I'm afraid I lost my temper and told her that I hadn't broken my leg, I had broken my neck! She reluctantly agreed to maintain visits once every 2 weeks to do my laundry until April when my daughter would be home from university. This never happened. She also told me to contact Social Services to take over. Of course, I didn't qualify because I had income—but only enough to pay regular bills and buy food. There was nothing left over to pay for help.

Based on Janet's experience in the Toronto area, home care, which is delivered through Community Care Access Centres, is not consistent across the board. It depends which of the original municipalities (before amalgamation) you reside in. At one point, the East York Home Care program ran out of money in the summer, but if you lived in the old boundaries of the City of Toronto, you were fine.

What Canada Can Learn from other Health Care Jurisdictions

Much like self-managed attendant care, a model that allows people leaving the hospital to pay whom they choose for care would make things much simpler and cheaper. In the United Kingdom, anyone who meets the qualification of disabled, be it from a spinal cord injury or cancer, is automatically given a $125 week allowance, tax-free. This amount is to pay for taxis, homemaking, and anything else the person wants. It does not have to be accounted for. Such a system could operate in Canada. For example, in Janet's case the grant would have continued for 6 months to a year with a review after that time. It would also allow people to use some of the funds to compensate family members who stop working to care for parents and children with disabilities.

The idea of allowing Canadians to access Employment Insurance (EI) to take care of relatives with disabilities is a start. But what about the Canadians who have been performing the role for many years already? What about their Canada Pension Plan contributions that have been forfeited to take care of a relative? What about all the people who aren't eligible because they were self-employed and not covered by EI? There are too many inconsistencies that make the current system unfair and inequitable.

Caregiving and the Role of Families and of Society

Dr. Murray Waldman comments:

We have families of patients in the hospital who are willing to do anything they possibly can short of taking care of mother! And they become the most adamant that—you're not working hard enough; she could do better; she should stay longer; and the degree of the stridency seems to be proportional to how far away they live. The son who lives in California is on the phone all the time screaming that we are not looking after his mother adequately, but when we suggest that he come into town and help out, of course he is far too busy. It is not his job. And I am not entirely sure what the answer to that is—we should be facing this as a society and asking, "What obligations do we have?"

One of the problems with home care issues is that it tends to be diagnosis-based rather than disability-based. Which is not sensible!

The obligation for the care of anyone who is disabled should not have to be hands-on. I think a wonderful system, which would help tremendously, would be to pay families who are taking loads off the system. For example, if you look after your mother at home, we (the government/Ministry of Health) will split the difference with you. The burden of care that way becomes shared and offers a bonus for the caregivers. At present,

altruism doesn't pay! Unfortunately, behaving selfishly
does pay!

In a report to the Ontario Ministry of Health in
September, 2000, the Ontario Brain Injury Association
states that, "In 1996, 7,983 people were admitted to
hospital with traumatic brain injury (TBI). This figure
does not include people with TBI who were examined in
the emergency ward or by their family physician and
sent home." The report also mentions that, in Ontario,
the total number is estimated at 17,000 per year. Of the
Ontario numbers, approximately 4,100 will die as a
result of brain injury, and many survivors will be left
with life-altering, long term disabilities. These
disabilities may be physical, cognitive, behavioural or a
combination of the three. There are many other non-
traumatic brain injuries from diseases such as
meningitis and from strokes and acquired brain injury,
which have become leading causes of disability.

Not only is respite care needed for caregivers
providing at-home care, but also funding for planned
respite care should be increased and augmented by a
plan for emergency respite care. This is critically
important when caregivers have medical emergencies
themselves or other dependents require medical
treatment. As caregivers age, there is going to be more
and more need for these services. Currently, respite care
funding is woefully inadequate.

The Romanow Commission on Health Care Reform

Although home care was not considered a medically
necessary service under medicare, all provinces and
territories recognize its value. But the variations across
the country are diverse and the amount individuals
have to pay varies. The Romanow Commission
recommended expansion of the term "medically
necessary" in the Canada Health Act to include services

provided other than by a hospital or physician. The Romanow Commission recommended that mental health, post-acute care and palliative (end-of-life) care be the first areas of home care to come under the Canada Health Act.

In the wake of the Romanow report, more money has been made available in recognition that home care needs to be included under the Canada Health Act. In both palliative and post-acute care, the need is expected to be relatively short-term and finite. But the home care and respite care needs of long term caregivers are really not being addressed. The idea is that the resources the provinces currently devote to these areas of health care can then be used to expand the long term care needs of people with disabilities or chronic illnesses. The question is, will this actually happen? Time will tell.

For nursing home care, programs among the provinces vary from extensive coverage in some areas to the provision of a monthly dollar amount for patients in others. There may be hourly limits on the amount of care and, in some areas, long term care may be the only option. Provision of supplies may be on a means-tested basis or for a limited time or for certain supplies only. For home rehabilitation, it varies from extensive services to none at all. British Columbia requires 12 months residency before individuals become eligible (perhaps to stop other Canadians from moving to a milder climate?), but other provinces require 3 months' residency. Several provinces require either co-payments or provide services only on a means-tested basis.

Close to 10% of New Brunswick's budget goes to health care; in Nunavut it is less than 2%. Across Canada, on average, 4 to 5% of the health care budget is spent on home care, with Ontario being average and Quebec well below. These disparities mean that Canadians with long term home care needs do look at moving to a province with a better delivery of home care services.

The Romanow Commission recommended funding (a) for case management to monitor the health of mental health patients, and (b) home intervention to assist and support clients during acute periods of disruptive behaviour. This support would also apply to patients with Alzheimer's disease and other similar conditions that need case management support.

The Romanow Commission's recommendations for post-acute home care would include case management, health professional services, and medication management for 14 days after discharge from acute care or 28 days if rehabilitation is needed for the specific condition. Currently, in many provinces, patients are discharged after some surgery, (such as gall bladder removal), on the same day. Although this surgery is less problematic than in earlier times, there is at present *no* follow up or home care.

According to the estimates in the Romanow Commission's report, only 5% of Canadians have access to palliative home care. Canadians in rural and remote locations and Canadians with disabilities have limited access to hospice palliative care. It has not been considered as a basic entitlement under medicare. The Romanow Commission recommends palliative home care for people with a prognosis of death within 6 months. This should include case management, pain and symptom relief, professional services, medication management, and counselling. And "respite care should also be provided where appropriate."

The federal government has agreed to fund a 5-year health reform fund transferring resources for health care to the provinces. As part of the 2003 First Ministers' Accord on Health Care Renewal, premiers addressed the issue of home care services and agreed to provide funding for short-term acute care, including acute community mental health and end-of-life (palliative) care. The minimum services to be provided will be determined by September 30, 2003, to be implemented through 2006. The expectation is that by

2006 the services *could* include nursing and professional services, pharmaceutical drugs and medical equipment and supplies, support for essential personal care needs, and assessment of client needs and case management.

In the same document, the Government of Canada agreed to implement a *compassionate care benefit* through the Employment Insurance Program "for those who need to temporarily leave their job to care for a gravely ill or dying child, parent or spouse." Unfortunately, this will assist people only in the short term and makes the assumption that people have been employed by employers, rather than being self-employed or business owners, or homemakers with their own families. In other words, this is a short term solution which ignores long term care giving needs.

The other element of the First Ministers' accord that applies here is the recognition of the need for catastrophic drug coverage, which is expected to be implemented in 2005-06.

Extended Health

Many extended health care plans have some coverage for physiotherapy, massage therapy, and the services of other practitioners. These plans vary enormously—from no coverage to several thousand dollars per year of benefit. Some policies include a long term care benefit as well as coverage for semi-private hospital rooms, prescription drugs, and dental costs. In many cases, though, the premiums for coverage after age 65 become prohibitive. Again, as with all insurance plans, understand what coverage you have and if necessary, purchase additional coverage to top up the basic benefit. (See Chapter 5, "Employee and Individual Benefits.")

Remember that if a disability is the result of a motor vehicle or workplace accident, or as a result of a tort claim (see Chapter 12, "When Can You Sue?") additional health care benefits such as physiotherapy, chiropractic, massage therapy, etc., will be part of the settlement or paid for automatically by the insurance company or agency.

Business owners who have set up personal health or extended health services plans can use these plans to claim up to $10,000 of medical expenses with no deductible. This is particularly useful for uncovered therapies and medical equipment that would otherwise have to be paid for directly. (See Chapter 10, "Disability and the Self-employed Small Business Person.")

Driving Test Issues

Some disabilities are *reportable* to the provincial Ministry of Transportation. This means that the attending physician must report the patient's diagnosis to the ministry. The reason for this is that some injuries or conditions may impair a person's ability to safely operate an automobile. Spinal cord injuries (even if the person is not permanently paralyzed), brain injury, stroke, and diagnosis of Alzheimer's, among others, will result in a request for an assessment of the person's driving ability. Failure to comply results in an automatic suspension of the person's driving licence.

In Ontario, this assessment is not a regular driving test. Instead, it is a series of assessments which includes medical reports, vision, cognitive, and reaction time tests as well as an on-road evaluation. The driving portion of the test is administered by an evaluator and the other portions by an occupational therapist. These same people also provide training on hands-only controls for people with paraplegia.

When the person does not perform to standard, sometimes all that is required is a few lessons to build confidence again.

Janet's story

Several other people I know had to take lessons in order to maintain their driver's licence. The "problem" was that they were driving too slowly—a logical result of awareness of their disability. In my case, I passed the test with flying colours and as a result, I have more confidence driving again than I would have had otherwise.

These assessments cost money—several hundred dollars and then more if lessons are required. (These costs can be claimed as a medical expense on your income tax return). It can easily cost someone $1,000-$2,000 to maintain their licence. These costs are not normally covered by extended health plans. Again, when the disability is covered by a motor vehicle, tort, or worker's compensation claim, these costs would be covered.

Allowing your driving licence to be suspended with the thought that you will get it back later is *not* a good idea. Having a suspended licence on your record could make getting auto insurance coverage again either very costly or impossible.

Cultural Issues

Cultural differences play a part in the individual's recovery. In some cultures, the attitude is, "Now that I'm sick or disabled my family have to take care of me." People who have this attitude may not participate in physiotherapy and occupational therapy or any of the other activities involved in rehabilitation.

One social worker interviewed for this book spoke about a couple who were immigrants to Canada. She asked them what happens in their country of origin if someone has a spinal cord injury. The response was that they go to nursing homes—they are not visible in the community. One particular client wanted this for her husband, but he adamantly refused to go to a nursing home. In fact, he wanted to move back into his own home with modifications. It is important to recognize how vital it is to ask the right questions of the family so that you understand where they're coming from and what their cultural influences are.

Some Innovations

Day Hospital
The cost of full-time in-hospital care is enormous. But, in most cases, in order to get the full range of rehabilitative services (from physiotherapy to psychological counselling, as well as learning to live with the disability), people with disabilities need to be *in-patients* rather than *out-patients*.

But there are people whose needs fall between those of in-patients and out-patients. Their injuries may be less severe or they may progress to the point where they do not require a hospital bed and can manage as out-patients for physiotherapy and occupational therapy. These people are short-changed if they do not get the same level of therapeutic service as in-patients, because they do not participate in the support system that tends to develop in the hospital, nor do they receive such intensive therapy and the opportunity to actually work on their own in the gym.

To address the needs of patients in this situation, the Toronto Rehabilitation Institute at the Lyndhurst Spinal Cord Centre has started a therapeutic program with the goal of providing services for patients who no longer require a hospital bed, but do require continuing intensive therapy. Not technically a "day" hospital, because there are no bathing facilities available, nevertheless the program offers a wide range of services including:
- Physiotherapy and occupational therapy
- nursing
- teaching

- services of a psychologist, social worker, and dietician
- wound and skin care
- seating clinic
- recreational services
- caregiver support
- other clinics for specific services
- out-patient follow-up

The Lyndhurst program offers priority to Lyndhurst patients and all out-patients must require two services to qualify for the program.

These innovative programs change the system so that people have the option of going home at night, if possible, to spend time with their families while maintaining their full rehabilitation program. This prevents people from leaving a rehabilitation facility too soon and forfeiting needed rehabilitation therapy, and ultimately increased function. Individuals still have the benefits of the support system without being an in-patient. It also saves money for the hospital!

Out-of-province Facilities

Not every province has the capacity to provide top-level post-acute care for its injured residents. Serious spinal cord injuries resulting in quadriplegia are not very common compared to strokes and heart attacks requiring rehabilitation. This is why some people in rehabilitation may need to receive care outside their home province, in order to receive specialzed treatment. This is particularly the case for people with spinal cord injuries. As might be expected, Ontario has many facilities for rehabilitation, (and spinal cord rehabilitation) in Toronto, Ottawa and London. In Quebec, there is the Centre de Rehabilitation and the Montreal Jewish General Hospital. There is a small rehabilitation unit in New Brunswick for spinal cord injuries. There are excellent rehabilitation facilities in

Alberta (Edmonton) and British Columbia (Vancouver). Other medical conditions that are more common than spinal cord injury will be handled in facilities in most major urban centres.

Provinces such as Newfoundland, Prince Edward Island, Nova Scotia, New Brunswick, Saskatchewan, and the Territories usually send serious, less common rehabilitation cases, such as spinal cord injury patients, out of province. When this is done, medicare in the patient's province of residence covers the costs for in-patient rehabilitation services. However, in most cases, travel costs for family members are not covered unless the patient has private insurance or, of course, if costs are being covered through a legal claim, motor vehicle insurance, or workers' compensation claim.

Janet's story

> *One of the important elements of rehabilitation is encouraging people to do as much for themselves as possible. And those things may be very small. I'll always remember Irv's excitement when he could hold and light his own cigarette; Jimmy's huge sense of accomplishment when, as a complete quadriplegic, he regained minimal movement in his right thumb so that he could use a regular electric wheelchair rather than the "sip-and-blow" type that he had been using. For me, it was not needing a nurse to dress and bathe me and going to the bathroom on my own.*
>
> *Dressing oneself, feeding oneself, bathing oneself, going to the bathroom unassisted mean so much. The dependency on others created by serious disease or an accident is one of the most devastating effects. After all, most of us don't even remember the time when we couldn't walk, dress ourselves and feed ourselves and perform all those other day-to-day tasks that people without disabilities take for granted. Being able to walk again is actually much lower down the list—*

wheels can replace legs and allow for movement unassisted by another person.

Vulnerability is another large issue. When you are unable to get out of bed unassisted, there is the recognition that if there is an emergency such as a fire, you are totally dependent on someone else to rescue you. The flight and fight response is alive and well and kicking (often heightened after a spinal cord injury), but you can do neither.

One of the major long term effects of disability is fatigue. Learning how to pace oneself is very important, but hard to do. When I feel good, I still tend to do too much and then have no energy the following day or two. But the fatigue issue can translate into other areas too. Employers, family, and friends often don't recognize the need for more frequent rest breaks, or that someone who looks and acts well can suffer devastating fatigue, and that the very effort of getting out of bed, bathing and making and eating breakfast can take 2 to 3 hours (after which you feel ready to go back to bed!) Nobody is looking for sympathy—just recognition of some limitations and support to allow us to do for ourselves everything that we can. And for the things that we need help with, to be done quietly and unobtrusively.

When disability hits while we are relatively young, especially at a time when we are used to being caregivers and not care recipients, the adjustment is hard. At the time of my accident, I still had a daughter at home. Although my children were older, I was still parenting them, not having them taking care of me. It was too soon! I felt overwhelmed by the support and caring of friends, colleagues, and clients—but I was supposed to be taking care of them! I think I shed more tears over that than anything else.

It is important that not just professional caregivers but friends, family and acquaintances be aware of these issues. When I was struggling to put on a jacket one time while still in a wheelchair, a well-meaning friend automatically rushed over to help—and got a very sharp response. It may take more time, and it is frustrating to watch someone struggle, but ninety-nine times out of a hundred, someone who needs help will ask for it. And you can always say, "Let me know if you want me to help." Then, let the person you are helping direct that assistance.

A friend of mine, who also learned to walk again, refuses to use a cane and often falls over while walking. He doesn't hurt himself, and can get up by himself. He was telling me about a man and his son who rushed over to help him one time after he had fallen, and he really snapped at the young son who was the first to reach him. Once he had recovered he explained that it was really important to him to be able to do this himself, it was fine to offer help, but to hold back unless wanted. It is a real problem though—we don't want people to stop being Good Samaritans (I wouldn't be here without them!) but learning the right approach is important.

Sometimes the response to unwanted assistance appears to be quite out of character or an "over-the-top" response with anger, physical, or verbal abuse. Remember, even young children, if you try to hurry them or help them when they don't want to be helped, often react very negatively. Over the years, we learn to let them do things for themselves as part of learning to become independent. Imagine the frustration, then, when these simple tasks have to be relearned, or even worse, when loss of function means ongoing dependency on others. Having regained most function, I know what I fear most is becoming dependent again—even at age 90! Independence and living independently are what people with disabilities want most.

SOURCES OF INFORMATION

The Romanow Commission on Health Care Information can be found at the following Web sites:

Health Canada www.hc-sc.gc.ca/english/care/romanow/
Canadian Health Services Research Foundation www.chsrf.ca
Canadian Health Coalition www.healthcoalition.ca

Recommended Reading:

From the Ashes of My Dreams, Ed Smith. Flanker Press, 2002
   A personal account of adventures and misadventures in
   hospitals and rehabilitation centres in Newfoundland and
   Ontario, following a motor vehicle accident.

RESOURCES

There are over 5,000 Web sites in Canada providing information and resources to Canadians with disabilities. The following are just a few of those resources. Web sites specific to chapter topics are included in the *Sources of Information* section at the end of each chapter.

FEDERAL GOVERNMENT INFORMATION SOURCES

Local telephone numbers for federal government offices can be found in the blue pages of your telephone book.

Human Resources Development Canada (HRDC)
www.hrdc.gc.ca

General enquiry number for Canada Pension Plan questions and application forms for CPP disability pension:
1-800-277-9914
To reach a live person, stay on the line and someone will eventually answer!

Canada Customs and Revenue Agency (CCRA)
www.ccra.gc.ca

PROVINCIAL GOVERNMENT INFORMATION SOURCES

Local telephone numbers can be found in the blue pages of your telephone book

Web sites

Alberta www.gov.ab.ca	Nova Scotia www.gov.ns.ca
British Columbia	Nunavut www.gov.nu.ca
www.gov.bc.ca	Ontario www.gov.on.ca
Manitoba www.gov.mb.ca	Prince Edward Island
New Brunswick	www.gov.pe.ca
www.gov.nb.ca	Quebec www.gouv.qc.ca
Newfoundland & Labrador	Yukon www.gov.yk.ca
www.gov.nf.ca	
Northwest Territories	
www.gov.nt.ca	

GENERAL DISABILITY LINKS

Enablelink www.enablelink.org

This site has lots of resources and listings of national, provincial, and local organizations for all disabilities. Information on everything from housing to injured workers.

The site is run by the *Canadian Abilities Foundation* which publishes the magazine, *Abilities*

General Contact Information:
The Canadian Abilities Foundation
340 College Street, Suite 650
Toronto, ON M5T 3A9
Ph: (416) 923-1885

Directory for accessibility (Ontario March of Dimes)
A one-stop resource of Ontario-based companies and organizations that provide services or assistance for people with disabilities. www.acessibilitydirectory.ca

People with Disabilities online
www.pwd-online.ca
(Federal government site)

Council of Canadians with Disabilities
www.ccdonline.ca

DISABILITY ORGANIZATIONS – SPECIFIC CONDITIONS/SERVICES

Most national organizations provide links to provincial organizations. Where there is no national organization, provincial links are provided here. Most of these sites provide many other links to other disability Web sites and related organizations, including international organizations. Where there is no national organization, provincial Web sites only are listed. Check your local telephone directory.

Active Living Alliance for Canadians with a Disability
104-720 Belfast Road,
Ottawa, Ont. K1G 0Z5
Tel: 1-800-771-0663
www.ala.ca

Alzheimer Society of Canada
1200-20 Eglinton Ave. West,
Toronto, Ont. M4R 1K8
Tel: 416-488-8772
www.alzheimer.ca

Association for the Neurologically Disabled of Canada
The A.N.D Centre
59 Clement Road
Etobicoke, Ontario
Canada M9R 1Y5
Telephone: 416-244-1992
www.and.ca

Brain Injury Associations
Alberta www.biaa.ab.ca
British Columbia
   www.brainassociation.com
Manitoba www.mts.net

New Brunswick (no Web site)
   Tel: 506-446-3696
Newfoundland and Labrador
   www.nbia.nf.ca
Nova Scotia www3.ns.
   sympatico.ca/bians1
Ontario www.obia.on.ca
Quebec www.aira.com
Saskatchewan
   www.sfn.saskatoon.sk.ca

Canadian Cancer Society
1639 Yonge Street,
Toronto, Ont. M4T 2W6
Tel: 416-488-5400
www.cancer.ca

Canadian Home Care Association
17 York Street, Suite 401
Ottawa, Ontario K1N 9J6
Phone: (613) 569-1585
www.cdnhomecare.on.ca

Canadian Mental Health Association
8 King Street East, Suite 810
Toronto ON M5C 1B5
Tel./Tél.: (416) 484-7750
www.cmha.ca

Canadian National Institute for the Blind
National Office
1929 Bayview Avenue
Toronto, ON M4G 3E8
Tel: 416-486-2500
www.cnib.ca

Canadian Paraplegic Association
230-1101 Prince of Wales Drive,
Ottawa, Ont. K2C 3W7
Tel: 1-800-720-4933
www.canparaplegic.org

Easter Seals / March of Dimes National Council
90 Eglinton Avenue East
Toronto, Ontario
M4P 2Y3
Phone: (416) 932-8382
www.esmodnc.org

Heart and Stroke Foundation of Canada
222 Queen Street, Suite 1402
Ottawa, ON K1P 5V9
Telephone (613)569-4361
www.heartandstroke.ca

Multiple Sclerosis Society of Canada
250 Bloor Street East,
Suite 1000
Toronto, Ontario M4W 3P9
Telephone: (416) 922-6065
www.mssociety.ca

Parkinson Society of Canada
4211 Yonge Street, Suite 316
Toronto, Ontario M2P 2A9
Toll Free: 1-800-565-3000
www.parkinson.ca

Red Cross
170 Metcalfe Street,
Suite 300
Ottawa, Ontario
K2P 2P2
Tel: (613)740-1900
www.redcross.ca

NATIONAL ADVOCACY & SUPPORT GROUPS

Most of these organizations have links to provincial and local chapters where applicable.

Canadian Association of Independent Living Centres (CAILC)
Promotes and enables the progressive process of citizens with disabilities to take responsibility for the development and management of personal and community resources.
1004 - 350 Sparks St.
Ottawa ON K1R 7S8

Phone: 613-563-2581
Web site: http://www.cailc.ca

Canadian Association of the Non-Employed

Carol Loveridge, Treasurer
c/o Workers Organizing Resource Centre
205 Notre Dame Ave.
Winnipeg MB R3B 1M8
Phone: 204-772-2952
Web site: www.pangea.ca

Canadian Health Coalition

The Canadian Health Coalition is dedicated to preserving and enhancing Canada's public health system for the benefit of all Canadians.
2481 Riverside Drive,
Ottawa, Ont. K1V 8X7
www.healthcoalition.ca

Canadian HIV/AIDS Legal Network

Educates about and promotes policy and legal responses to HIV infection and AIDS that respect human rights.
C.P. les Atriums
P.O. Box 32018
Montréal QC H2L 4Y5
Phone: 514-451-5457
Web site: www.aidslaw.ca

Canadian Injured Workers' Alliance

Reinforces and strengthens the work of local, territorial and provincial injured workers' groups, provides training and education resources and provides a forum for exchanging information and experiences.
P.O. Box 3678
237 Camelot Street.
Thunder Bay, ON
P7B 6E3
Phone: (807) 345-3429
Web site: www.ciwa.ca

Council of Canadians with Disabilities (CCD)
Improves status of persons with disabilities through
monitoring federal legislation as it impacts on people with
disabilities.
926 - 294 Portage Ave.
Winnipeg MB R3C 0B9
Phone: 204-947-0303
Web site: www.pcs.mb.ca

Court Challenges Program of Canada
Provides financial assistance for important court cases that
advance language and equality rights guaranteed under
Canada's constitution.
Contact: Director
616 - 294 Portage Ave.
Winnipeg MB R3C 0B9
Phone: 204-942-0022
Web site: www.ccppcj.ca

DAWN Canada
The DisAbled Women's Network of Canada is affiliated with
the provincial organizations of DAWN. DAWN is dedicated to
research, define the needs and concerns of women with
disabilities and designing programs to meet those needs. This
Web site contains feature articles and information about
ordering DAWN publications.
P.O. Box 22003
Brandon, MB R7A 6Y9
Phone: 204-726-1406
Web site: www.dawncanada.net

Injured Workers Online
A Web site which hosts a collaboration of injured workers,
trade unionists, community activists and doctors working to
improve the treatment of people with work-related
injuries/illnesses.
Web site: www.injuredworkers.org

National Institute of Disability Management and Research
Committed to reducing the human, social and economic cost
of disability to workers, employers and society through
education, training and research.

3699 Roger Street
Port Alberni, BC
Phone: (250) 724-4344
Web site: www.nidmar.ca

Rick Hansen Institute / Man in Motion Foundation

5th Floor, 520 West 6th Avenue
Vancouver, BC, Canada
V5Z 1A1 Phone: 604-876-6800
Web site: www.rickhansen.com

SCIPILOT

Spinal Cord Injured Peer Technology Information Library on
Technology
This site has firsthand accounts and advice from wheelchair
users on equipment funding and related issues.
www.scipilot.com

PUBLICATIONS

Disability Research Bulletin

Published by the Office for Disability Issues,
Human Resources Development Canada
Available on their Web site www.hrdc.gc.ca

Canadian Disability News

74 Mayfair Crescent,
Brampton, Ontario L6S 3N4
Tel: 905-792-9889
Subscription cost $25 yearly
www.signersnetwork.com

Abilities Magazine

Canadian Paraplegic Association
230-1101 Prince of Wales Drive,
Ottawa, Ont. K2C 3W7
Tel: 1-800-720-4933
www.canparaplegic.org

INDEX